LIFE BEYOND KETO

TASTY LOW CARB RECIPES TO SHARE WITH FRIENDS AND FAMILY

Mary Anne Young

CABIN FEVER PRESS

ISBN: 978-1984268648

Photos by Mary Anne Young
Book design and editing by David Haywood Young

CONTENTS

Vegetables

137

Poultry

183

Beef 215

Pork and Seafood 251

Beverages 273

Afterword 287

Why and How

WELCOME TO MY second cookbook!
   My first cookbook, "Grain Free Haven: The Cookbook", is full of recipes I converted from those traditionally made with grains. The idea was to give people a way to fill the holes in their grain free journey, left by memorable foods from their past.

This second book continues the grain free and sugar free trend of the first, but from a different perspective. It focuses on gatherings we all participate in, whether it is with family, friends, or in our communities. It focuses on dishes that can be shared or multiplied, made at the last minute or in advance for quick serving.

How did my family come to avoid grains and sugar? Here is a summary…

Many years ago my husband discovered, after experiencing a notable and debilitating illness, that he is highly sensitive to gluten. Further, gluten free grains did not do much to help his digestion or gastrointestinal tract. Too much information, maybe, but considering he was (hopefully) less than halfway through his life, there were many years ahead of eating. We had to figure out a long-term health strategy.

Given the occurrences of cancer, diabetes and dementia in both our family histories, we decided the best direction for our journey was excluding grains and sugar. This approach does not solve all problems, and to be frank, we have fallen off the wagon here and there over the years. Regardless, it was undeniable that we saw improvements in our health when we stayed on the wagon.

Another inspiration to exclude grains and sugar was our kids. Our daughter genetically inherited the potential to develop the same health problems we were trying to avoid, so it was an easy decision to include her in our journey. Our two adopted sons' family medical history at the very least include heart and cancer issues, and their diets prior to joining our family were not very balanced. As they get older we do what we can to encourage them to make healthy eating decisions for themselves by being good examples. We continue to work to be good examples for them, and hope that a minimum of grains and sugar in their childhood will make a lifelong positive impact, even if they eat more "junk" when older, and away from home.

You may have a few questions about this book. Here are a few answers.

Where is the nutrition information?

I thought about including nutrition details for the recipes, but I decided to exclude them. Why? Because ingredient nutrition info can vary depending on brands and fat/nonfat versions. I didn't feel they could accurately represent what was actually made. Also, there are so many apps out there people already rely on, especially those following ketogenic or diabetic diets, I didn't want to muddy the proverbial water.

But, where are the desserts?

You will have to get the first cookbook for those. What I discovered as we moved forward without grains or sugar, was that desserts took a smaller and smaller role in our meals. If the kids want something sweet we make sure raw fruits are available, like grapefruit, berries and watermelon. There are definitely still desserts at our friend and family gatherings, but we leave them for other people to provide. We just stopped focusing on them, so there aren't many more tried and true recipes in our repertoire that I have not already shared. As for sweet, check out the Beverages section, for it has some fun treats!

What the heck is stevia?

When sweet is added to a recipe we rely on fruit or pure, concentrated stevia powder. We have tried a lot of different sweeteners over the years, some of which have since been shown to cause more problems than sugar. The plant based fiber supplement represented in pure stevia powder is the healthiest option we know of to add sweet to a dish without raising the glycemic index. It has been used in South America as a sweetener for over a thousand years, and was finally approved as a dietary supplement in the US in the 1990s. Today it is an accepted and safe ingredient in products available in the US. One more item about stevia: any time I use stevia in a recipe I also include the equivalent for pure cane sugar. For those of you who use sugar, or another type of sweetener, it is the best way I know of to reflect the amount of sweetness added.

What about the family and friends who eat grains and sugar?

Not everyone is invested in avoiding grains and sugars. I know some people cook grain free or sugar free for themselves, while serving something else to friends and family. All the recipes I am sharing store well or freeze well, with the exceptions of Dressings and Sauces. I know from experience that eating in a manner that excludes certain foods means it is sometimes tough to stay on track, so having leftovers easily available is important. Go ahead and cook extra, putting away leftover servings for times when you need it quickly. When taking dishes to gatherings I have found that bringing something I can eat will ensure there is something I can eat! Also, I have found that as a hostess I can prepare grain based or starchy sides, served along with pretty much any of my recipes (especially those with sauces), but I don't have to eat them. I will stop here and leave the rest to you. My family and friends spent a lot of time in the kitchen and at tables to test and create these recipes. We also accumulated a ton of memories, and in the process we hope we have extended our lives through the healing power of food. I hope this book helps you on your journey!

Why do some of the pictures have carby foods included?

Because we feed multiple people. The reality of our household is that some eat rice, for instance, and some don't. We rarely serve it, and usually offer the option of riced cauliflower and/or rice. We may also put something like corn on the cob on the table. It is one of the aspects of feeding family and friends—people eat different things, and we try to recognize that fact on our table.

DEDICATION

WHEN IT COMES to family and friends there are three ladies who made a huge impact on how I see the world, so this book is dedicated to all three, for they cannot be separated.

My mom, Joanne Ward, passed on the deep family bond she developed when growing up in rural Tennessee. Her constant support and efforts to keep our family bonded and in touch are a quintessential example of making family a priority.

My mother-in-law, Sherry Young, has been in my life since the age of eight. Besides her three children, she has a slew of children (now adults) who see her as a second mother. I am one of them and cherish how she has influenced my life.

My oldest friend and now sister-in-law, Kelley Young, is the third lady. She has been the calm in so many of my storms. Feeling in sync with someone else, whether in the same room or thousands of miles away, adds certain levels of peace and contentment to my world. I blame Kelley for helping me experience those levels for the past four decades.

Thanks ladies! I love you so very much!

APPETIZERS
&
SNACKS

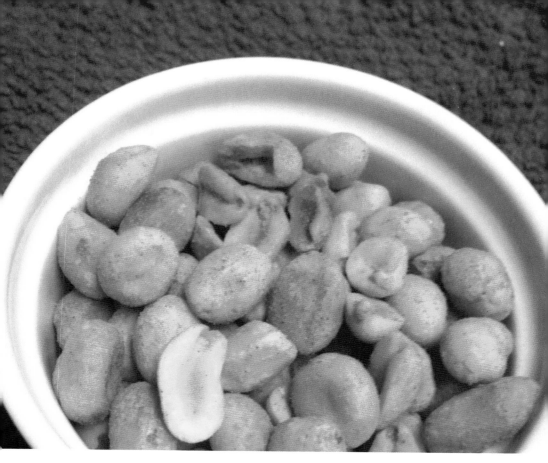

4 cups roasted, salted peanuts*
1/3 cup coconut oil, melted
1 tablespoon ground turmeric
1 teaspoon ground cinnamon
1 teaspoon garlic powder
1 teaspoon ginger powder
2 teaspoons ground cumin
1 teaspoon ground white pepper
1 teaspoon red chili powder
½ teaspoon ground clove

*If you want to start with raw blanched or unblanched peanuts, it is quite simple. Spread 2 cups of shelled peanuts on a tray, place into 350 degree oven for ten minutes. Stir halfway through and let cool before continuing the recipe. If you do two trays at the same time just switch oven shelves halfway through. Add salt to seasoning paste to taste, as well.

Curry Peanuts

If you ever have a hankering for Indian peanut curry dishes, you will like these peanuts. A handful of the spice and protein makes for a filling, satisfying snack.

Prep Time: 5 minutes

Cook Time: 20 minutes

Servings: 32 1-ounce servings

Preheat oven to 300 degrees. Line two medium sized shallow baking sheets with foil.

In a large bowl, combine coconut oil and spices into a paste (add salt to taste if you started with unroasted nuts). Add nuts and toss until coated. Spread nuts on the sheets in a single layer. Bake for ten minutes.

Remove sheets from oven and toss nuts. Return nuts to oven, making sure to switch sheet levels in oven if baking more than one sheet at a time. Bake for an additional 5–10 minutes until slightly browned.

Remove from oven and let sit until completely cooled. Store in an airtight container.

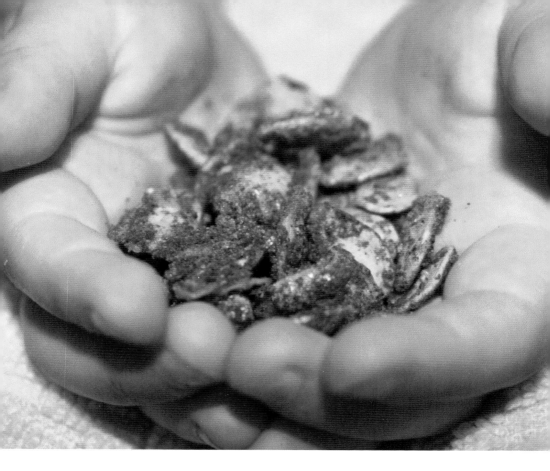

1 teaspoon turmeric
1 teaspoon garlic powder
2 teaspoon ground cinnamon
1 teaspoon chili powder
¼ teaspoon pure stevia powder (optional)
1 tablespoon olive oil
1½ cups squash seeds (pumpkin,
 spaghetti squash, acorn squash, etc)

Roasted Squash Seeds

This recipe, although it includes stevia, is surprisingly savory, but helps balance the flavors. It is a great way to fully utilize the seeds of squash that are otherwise so often discarded.

Prep Time: 5 minutes (plus 30 minutes drying time)

Cook Time: 30 minutes

Servings: 12 1-ounce servings

Preheat oven to 250 degrees. Separate seeds from sinew and set out to dry on a tray for at least half an hour. Don't worry about rinsing them or getting every strand–any squash left on the seeds helps to enhance and carry the flavors.

In a small bowl combine spices and stevia, then add the oil and stir. Add seeds and toss until coated. Spread seeds on a cookie sheet, making sure they are spread out as much as possible.

Toast for about 30 minutes, until dried out and crispy. Remove from oven and let cool. Store in an airtight container.

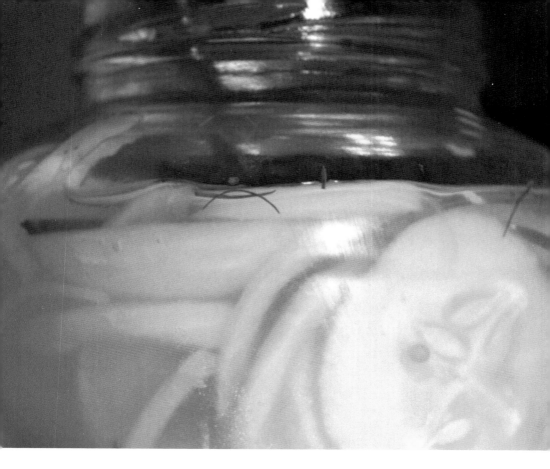

1 large cucumber, peeled
1–2 cups white vinegar (substitute half the
  vinegar with distilled water if you want
  less tang)
½ white onion, julienne sliced
2 teaspoons salt
5 sprigs fresh dill
4 - 6 cloves garlic, chopped
1 tablespoon mustard seeds

Refrigerator Dill Pickles

When I was a kid we had a garden in the back yard. We always grew tomatoes and sunflowers. We usually included zucchini and cucumbers. Needless to say, we ate a lot of fresh vegetables during the summer.

Sometimes I looked forward to the gardening–finding fruit and veggies ready to pick or grabbing some of the more elusive weeds while the plants matured. Other times I was not so eager to be a gardener–breaking up all the clods of dirt after they clumped over the winter, or clearing out all the dead plants when autumn came.

One thing my mom always did with some of our cucumber crop was make refrigerator pickles. For months there would be at least one jar of pickles in the fridge door–we would come in from playing outside (or gardening) and pinch a few cold, tart slices as a snack. They never lasted very long, which was good, since the simple preparation did not include any heating or effort to sterilize or pasteurize in the process.

A wonderful snack during summer or anytime!

Prep Time: 10 minutes

Cook Time: 24 hours of chilling

Servings: 12

Sanitize glass jar (at least 1 quart size with tight fitting lid) Slice cucumbers into coins, about 1/8 inch thick. Set aside. In a glass jar with tight fitting lid combine vinegar and spices. Put lid on jar and shake. Add cucumber to jar, making sure the slices are not sticking together. Secure lid on jar again and shake vigorously, encouraging the spices to spread out among the slices. Chill for at least 24 hours before eating and store in refrigerator.

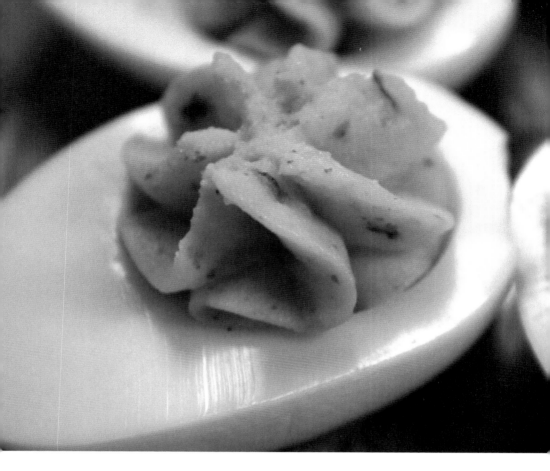

12 large eggs
½ teaspoon raw horseradish
1 teaspoon yellow or stone ground mustard
½ teaspoon curry powder
1-2 tablespoons mayonnaise (in Sauces) or plain
   yogurt
2 tablespoons green onion, finely chopped
Paprika for garnish (optional)

*Instead of cake decorating equipment you can use a strong plastic bag. Fill bag with yolk mixture and pack it down into one corner. Snip the corner of the bag with scissors, making about a 1/8 inch to 1/4 inch opening. Squeeze mixture through opening into egg white halves.

Deviled Eggs

From what I can tell, deviled eggs got their name from being spicy, as in full of flavor, and almost evil in their ability to tempt. Even the ancient Romans were known to partake of them.

Some people more devout than myself are wont to call them angel eggs, but there is nothing angelic about these babies. The horseradish gives them an tasty bite at the end, but can be left out if it does not work for you…

Prep Time: 30 minutes (plus 30 minutes chilling eggs)

Cook Time: 1 hour for chilling final eggs

Servings: 24 halves

Fill a large pot with about 4 inches of water. Place over high heat on stovetop and bring to a boil.

With a slotted spoon gently place eggs, one at a time, into the boiling water. Lower heat to maintain a simmer and cook eggs for 10 minutes until hard boiled. If using an Instant Pot, you can pressure eggs for three minutes and do Quick Release.

Remove pan from heat and tip to let hot water run out while cold water runs into the pot, gradually replacing hot water with cold and shaking the pan to crack the shells. Let set for about five minutes then peel. Peels should easily come off the eggs at this point.

After peeling let the eggs cool completely. When cold, slice eggs in half lengthwise and carefully remove yolks, placing them in a small bowl, while avoiding any damage to the whites. Arrange egg whites on serving dish.

Add all remaining ingredients to egg yolks and combine well. Take care to only use as much mayonnaise (in Sauces) or yogurt as needed to thin out the mixture, but stop short of making the mixture runny. It should be thick enough to hold shape, similar to cake frosting.

Place egg yolk mixture into cake decorating bag with a large decorating tip*. Fill egg whites with yolk mixture, using any kind of swirl or twist motion to make them pretty. Chill until time to serve. Sprinkle with paprika, optionally.

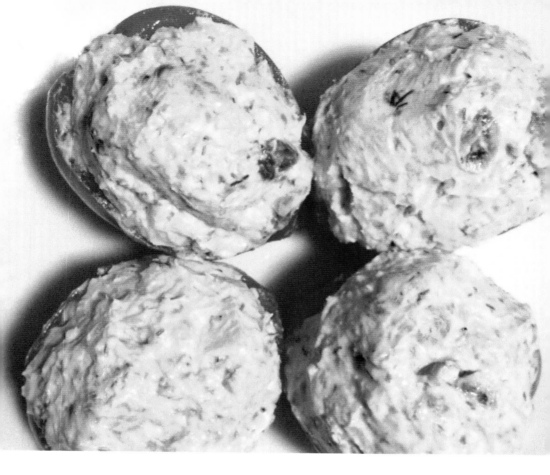

1 cup cream cheese, room temperature
½ cup sour cream
4 ounces smoked salmon, roughly chopped
1 garlic clove, crushed
1 teaspoon fresh dill, chopped (and a bit more for optional garnish)
2 celery stalks
5 large cherry tomatoes, or small salad tomatoes
5–10 slices sharp white cheddar cheese

Smoked Salmon Spread Crudite

This simple recipe for crudité can be adjusted to accommodate all types of diets and give variety to a meal, either before or during– even make them a meal on their own. Change up the vegetables and cheeses–pretty much anything you can cut in half and fill or top (carrots, cucumbers, olives, pickles).

Of course, crisped bread or crackers would work too! I hope you enjoy this easy appetizer and use your extra time to spend with your loved ones, because when it is all said and done, the people are what give you purpose.

Prep Time: 30 minutes (plus 1 hour chilling time for filling)

Cook Time: 20 minutes to use filling

Servings: 30

Whisk together cream cheese and sour cream. Add salmon and garlic, folding it into the cheese mixture until well combined. Chill for about an hour. While the spread chills prepare the serving bases.

Clean celery stalks, peel off tough strings and cut into 2 inch sticks. Clean tomatoes and slice in half lengthwise, scooping out the seeds and meat and place cut side down to dry. Slice cheese into 1 inch squares, making them thick enough to pick up and take a few bites out of, but thin enough not to over cheese the bites.

Spread the spread (heh) on all the bases, taking time to form it to complement the shape of the base–round the top like a tomato, curve the spread within the crevice of the celery, and a mound with some random irregularities to soften the edges of the cheese slices.

Garnish with more dill if you please. Serve immediately or chill until time to serve.

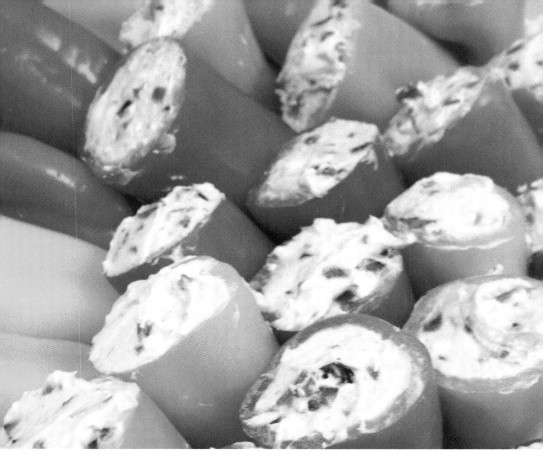

24 raw small sweet peppers, multicolored
8 ounces cream cheese, room temperature
6 ounces goat cheese, room temperature
1 tablespoon wasabi paste or horseradish (optional)
2 tablespoons lemon juice
½ cup chopped black olives
4 green onions, chopped
2 garlic cloves, finely diced
1 teaspoon salt

Stuffed Sweet Peppers

When we have a house full of visitors I like having the fridge full of ready to eat snacks and sides to accommodate everyone's diets, preferences and cravings. Being able to pull out a variety of snacks to fill people up between excursions and sit down meals is so nice.

Some people may disagree, but each sweet pepper color does have a different flavor. I have stuffed them before with milder cheese filling, but we were expecting visitors who like a bite to their food, so the addition of wasabi paste was perfect to go with the smooth cheeses and crispy peppers. The filling went well with all the pepper flavors and they disappeared quickly during snack times.

Prep Time: 20 minutes

Cook Time: 1 hour for chilling

Servings: 24

In a medium bowl combine the cream cheese, goat cheese and wasabi. Fold in the olives, onions, garlic, lemon juice, and salt. Remove the top stem portion from all the peppers, scraping out the membrane and seeds with a small spoon. Using a spoon or piping bag with round tip, fill each pepper with the cheese mixture. Chill until ready to serve.

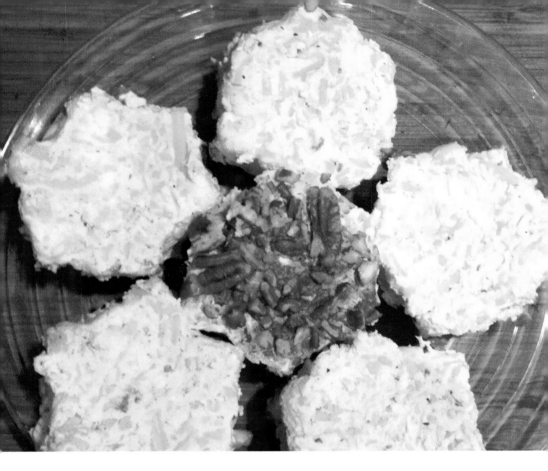

2½ cups sharp cheddar cheese, grated and at
  room temperature
8 ounces cream cheese, room temperature
4 ounces goat cheese, room temperature
½ teaspoon red chili flakes
1 teaspoon ground cumin
1 cup toasted pecans, chopped (optional)

Cheese Balls

If you look closely at the ingredients of various cheese balls available at the grocery, there is a curiously large amount of them containing sugar, soy and wheat. As frequent cheese consumers, we found it logical to make our own and avoid the sugar and grains. This one is simple and can be molded in all kinds of ways. The cheese mixture is extremely versatile and delicious!

Prep Time: 30 minutes

Cook Time: 1 hour chilling time

Servings: 32 (1 ounce each)

Using a mixer with whisk attachment combine together cream cheese, goat cheese, chili flakes and cumin. Add cheddar cheese and stir together with other cheeses. The mixture may be a bit stiff if you don't have a strong mixer, so mixing it together with your hands (like I often do) works great.

Drop cheese mixture onto a piece of cling wrap that is twice the size of the mixture. Using the cling wrap mold the cheese into the desired shape–sphere, log, oval, etc.

You can also use a gelatin mold or other shape to form the cheese. If desired, roll shaped cheese in pecans and gently press them into the cheese. Chill at least an hour before serving with vegetables or crackers.

NOTE: There is no added salt, because the strong cheeses typically give sufficient tartness. If you choose to use less strong cheeses you may want to add salt to the mixture.

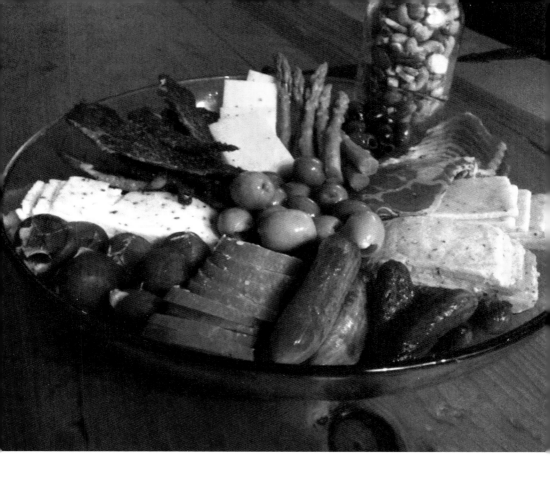

Dry coppa, pastrami or prosciutto
Dry Salami
Beef Jerky
Roasted Chestnuts
Garlic Stuffed Olives
Jalapeno Stuffed Olives
Mustard (suggest stone ground and
  horseradish style)
Dry Roasted Mixed Nuts
Specialty Cheeses, sliced
Pickled Asparagus
Pickles
Dried Fruit (optional)

Yule Platter

Every year on winter solstice, also traditionally called Yule, we have a family party. Especially during our winter time in Alaska the solstice was a big turning point–the shortest day of the year is the beginning of longer days and the approximate midpoint of chilly winter weather. More accurately the midpoint in locations further south…

Regardless of the weather, there is definitely a shortage of light. One way we celebrate Yule each year is to have a simple meal, made up of preserved foods that require little or no cooking. We don't do much of the preserving ourselves, but work off the labors of others. We smoke some jerky, onion, garlic and cheese, while other items like pickled veggies, cured meats and nuts are also added to the platter. We snack from the platter while sipping something bubbly–champagne for me, beer for my guy, and bubbly water for the kids.

It makes for a winter celebration we appreciate for its simplicity before the hustle and bustle of Christmas Eve and Day, which are full of our childhood traditions we are passing on to our kids. The simple celebration reminds us that the world is hibernating under the bare branches, blustery winds and wet ground. A time to ponder during a more sedate time of year when much of the natural world sleeps. Since there is not much recipe involved, here is a list of suggested items for your platter.

Prep Time: 20 minutes

Cook Time: 0

Servings: varies (plan on 4-8 ounces of cheese/meat per person)

Arrange ingredients in a pretty way on large platter. Offer and provide bubbly and/or fermented beverages. Eat, drink, be merry. Don't feel guilty about the ease of this dinner, for more complicated ones are bound to be on the horizon.

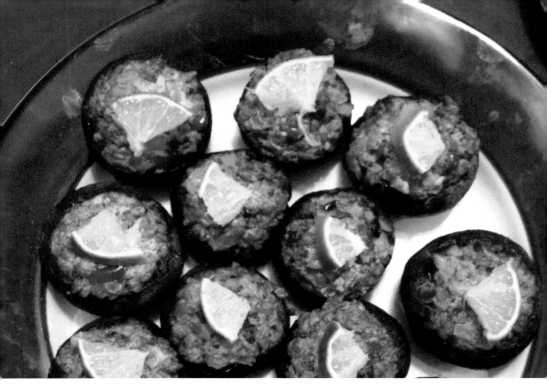

12 baby Portabello mushrooms
2 garlic cloves, finely diced
¼ medium white onion, finely diced
12 kalamata olives, pitted and finely chopped
3 slices of bacon, cooked crisp and crumbled
4 quarters marinated artichoke hearts, finely
  chopped
1 cup crumbled feta cheese
8-10 fresh basil leaves, chopped
½ teaspoon ground oregano
½ lime, juiced
2 tablespoon extra virgin olive oil
½ cup chicken broth
Salt to taste
Lime, thinly cut into slices and quartered
  (garnish)

Prep Time: 35 minutes

Cook Time: 30 minutes

Servings: 12

Kelley's Killer Stuffed Mushrooms

Have you ever felt like you are being watched? I did one day. I was sitting on my mom's patio and suddenly felt like I was being observed, with the strong need to figure out what was doing it. No people. No pets. A few birds were out there, but they were busy with the feeders.

In the end I decided it was the basil. Tall, healthy stalks rising out of a huge pot, with big, bright green leaves soaking up the morning sun. They were leaning slightly in my direction, so the little leaves at the very tips of the stalks worked like Cyclops' eyes….

I decided the only way to rid myself of the paranoia was to use some basil. It wants me to, right? A functional plant that just happens to be pretty, too?

I call them Kelley's Stuffed Mushrooms because my sister in law Kelley likes all things Greek. The ingredients have a leaning in the Greek direction, and they would be consumed at her house. Besides all that, she is one of the most awesome people on the planet.

Remove stems from mushrooms. With a small spoon scrape out brown gills from each mushroom cap, making more room for the stuffing. Finely chop the stems and scrapings.

In a large skillet over medium heat add the oil. When the oil is hot, add onion and garlic. Cook until onions soften but not yet browning. Add the chopped stems, olives, bacon, artichoke hearts, basil and oregano. Stir occasionally until stems are soft and combined with the other ingredients. Add feta to the pan and stir until it is melted and combined. Remove pan from heat, add juice from the half lime and stir.

Preheat oven to 375 degrees.

Divide stuffing among the mushroom caps, placing stuffed caps in a 9×12 inch baking dish. Slowly pour the broth in the pan, making a shallow pool under the caps. Place pan in oven and bake for 30 minutes, until mushrooms sweat and shrink. Remove from oven and let sit for about five minutes. Garnish with small lime slices (to be squeezed and juice sprinkled on top of each mushroom before eating) and serve.

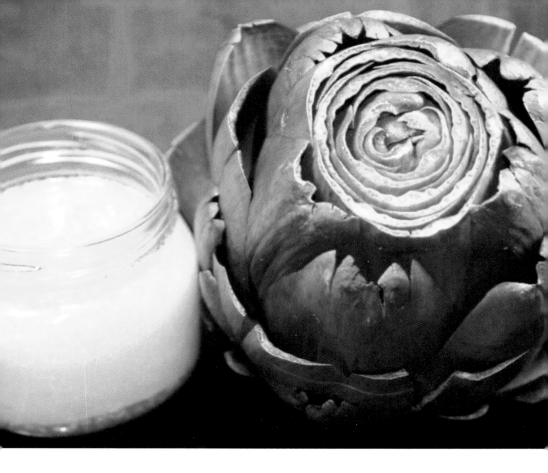

2 large, whole artichokes
4–6 cups water
3 tablespoons plus 1 teaspoon lemon juice
1 tablespoon plus ½ teaspoon salt
1 teaspoon black pepper
½ cup butter
1 clove garlic, crushed
½ cup mayonnaise (in Sauces)

Steamed Artichokes

I was about eight when I first remember eating an artichoke. My parents steamed a few. They set them up on plates with small bowls of aioli and melted butter for dipping. Here I was at the kitchen counter looking at this beautiful, yet also ugly green thing with little spikes on the ends of the leaves. I was supposed to eat it?

Mom and dad had a rule about food. You had to try everything. You didn't have to like it–liver, creamed turkey, coconut–but you gotta try it.

They showed me and my brother how to hold the prickly end and use our lower front teeth to scrape the meat off the tender end. I fell in love for the very first time. The meat had a gentle flavor, almost overwhelmed by the the dipping options of aioli and butter. The closer to the heart we got the more tender and sweet the meat.

Dad then showed us how to carefully scrape off the bristly choke to reveal succulent mouthfuls of the heart. The meat was not very filling and it took a bit of effort to get every bite, but what a treat!

Time warp forward about 12 years. My brother and I are sitting at his kitchen table in Austin. He had cooked about a half dozen artichokes in his back yard smoker. The leaf tips were brown and wrinkled, but the meat inside each leaf was soft, having been tickled with flavor from the smoking process.

We spent what must have been hours catching up with each others' lives and scraping the meat off every single artichoke leaf. The result was a lovely afternoon, an impressive pile of meat and hearts, and plans to make soup. The soup was simple–with all our efforts of the afternoon, all we had left to do was add garlic, cream and butter, then simmer for a bit. We continued talking while relishing every spoonful of soup. The cream of artichoke soup became yet another fond memory of mine closely tied to food.

Here is a simple method for preparing artichokes on the stovetop and enjoy sharing them with a crowd and some dipping sauces: (next page)

Prep Time: 20 minutes

Cook Time: 45 minutes

Servings: 4-6, shared

Cut off stem of artichoke just below the leaves until it sits level. Use kitchen scissors to clip off the tips of the larger, tougher leaves that have pulled away from the artichoke.

In a deep pot with steamer basket add the water (it should come right to the bottom of where the steamer basket will sit), 2 tablespoons of the lemon juice, 1 tablespoon of the salt and all the black pepper.

Bring water to a boil and add steamer basket, placing artichokes stem down in the basket, and cover. If artichokes cannot stand upright there are two alternatives: 1) they can be steamed laying on their sides, but should be flipped halfway through cooking, or 2) place the artichoke stem down, but use foil to cover and seal in the steam and hold them upright. Cover and return to boil.

Turn down heat to medium-low, but make sure the water continues to gently boil. Steam for 30–45 minutes. You will need less time if the artichokes are smaller, or more time if they are huge. The artichoke is ready when the center of the stem gives easily to a knife.

In a small sauce pan add butter, 1 tablespoon lemon, garlic and ½ teaspoon salt. Melt over medium-low heat until butter is melted and bubbly. Transfer butter to a small serving bowl for dipping.

In another small bowl stir together 1 teaspoon lemon juice with the mayonnaise. Add salt to taste.

Serve artichokes along with the two dipping sauces.

To eat the artichokes, peel off leaves and dip the pulled off end in your sauce of choice. Use your lower front teeth to scrape meat off then inside of each leaf. It helps to have an empty bowl nearby to collect the leaves when you finish with them. As you get closer to the heart the leaves will become smaller and more tender. You will be able to eat most of the leaf, carefully avoiding the prickly tips.

When you finally get to the bristly choke, take a spoon and scrape off the bristles, revealing the heart. Slice the heart and base and cut it into bite-size pieces. Dip and enjoy!

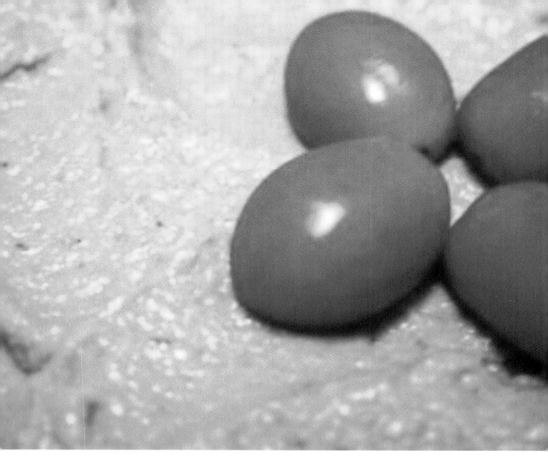

2 cups chicken broth
1 medium head cauliflower
2 cups chopped broccoli
1 small onion
2 celery stalks, trimmed and chopped
1 carrot, chopped (can be excluded for lower
   carbohydrate content)
2 cloves garlic
Salt and Pepper to taste

Vegetable Hummus

To reduce the number of carbohydrates typically found in hummus I came up with a way to make kinda-hummus, using veggies. I can use it where I would otherwise put chickpea based hummus, with fewer carbs while keeping the fiber content high.

The vegetable proportions can vary depending on what you have in the fridge, but keeping the cauliflower at about half the bulk will help obtain the hummus consistency.

Prep Time: 15 minutes

Cook Time: 45 minutes

Servings: 30 (1 ounce each)

Combine broth, garlic and vegetables in a large pot. Cook over medium high heat until boiling. Reduce heat and simmer for 30-45 minutes until all the vegetables are soft. Let cool until safe to transfer.

Using a strainer or slotted spoon, separate the veggies from the liquid. Purée the vegetables until smooth, all at once or in batches, using a blender, food processor or stick blender.

Add some of the cooking liquid only if the vegetables are too thick to purée. The vegetables will be pretty wet, so you probably won't need the liquid.

Serve warm or cold as a spread, dip or plating base for meats and other vegetables, as you would hummus.

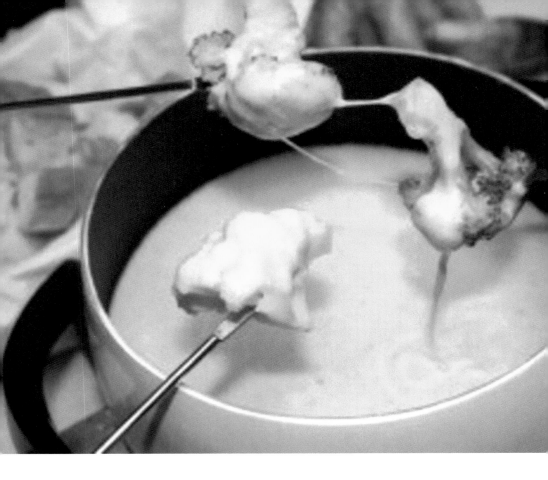

Prep Time: 2 hours day before serving, 1 hour day of serving

Cook Time: 2 hours during the meal

Servings: Varies - recommended quantities per person noted below

Fondue

Is it French or Swiss in origin? I don't know. The evolution in America of fondue is such a different animal compared to the simple cheese fondue I found to be served in Europe. Way back in the '80s, my family would join forces with other families and have fondue parties. At the time it was a throwback to the 1960s, when my parents stocked up on fondue sets. Regardless of when it peaked in popularity or where it first happened, it is still a fun time with abundant and delicious food.

The following recipes account for feeding seven people, since our most recent fondue party included as many guests. The meal called for a lot of preparation, but most of it can be done the day before, and makes for quick set up when it is actually time to eat. I pulled everything out of the refrigerator (yes, even the meats) about 45 minutes to an hour before serving so things were cool but not chilly.

Check out the Sauces section of this cookbook for sauces to serve with the oil and broth fondues: hollandaise sauce, chimichurri, mayonnaise with added garlic and lemon, lemon ginger sauce (see below). You can also use salad dressings, mustards, cocktail and tartar sauces.

I served the cheese fondue when people were first arriving and standing around in the kitchen, then served the oil and broth fondues at the table with all the sauces. Any sauces that inspire you can be served. Your meat, your party!

I did not even start preparing and melting the chocolate fondue until the table was cleared of the oil and broth. It was quick to do and a fun dessert.

And remember, you can always serve just one kind of fondue as an appetizer or single meal course. Your pot, your rules!

Cheese Fondue

    2 garlic cloves, cut in half
    1 cup dry white wine*
    8 ounces Gruyere cheese, shredded
    8 ounces Havarti cheese, shredded
    2 ounces Kerrygold Dubliner cheese, shredded (can substitute

a dry cheese, like romano)
1 tablespoon lemon juice
1 tablespoon Kirsch or brandy*
½ teaspoon nutmeg
½ teaspoon paprika
Black Pepper (optional)
Handful of cubed bread per person (can use grain free bread
   or pork rinds as substitutes)
Vegetables (can also used with Broth Fondue)

The measurements for wine and cheese should be enough, but you may want to have a little more on hand to adjust the consistency if needed. Add more cheese if it's too liquid, add more wine if it's too thick.

I have found that if you mix the cheese fondue on the stovetop or electric fondue pot about an hour before serving, then turn it off, but then start to reheat about ½ hour before serving, it makes for quick setup when guests first arrive.

To begin preparation, rub the garlic inside the fondue pot then discard. Pour the white wine and lemon juice into the pot and turn on the burner. Let the wine and lemon juice warm up without boiling. Reduce heat and add the shredded cheese. With a wooden spoon, mix well and stir regularly. Add the Kirsch or brandy, and add remaining ingredients to the pot. Add pepper to taste. Adjust consistency with additional wine or cheese.

Dip bite size pieces of bread, pork rinds or vegetables. Let the freshly dipped pieces cool off for a few seconds before enjoying. Extra liquid may be needed after the fondue is half gone because it thickens as time passes.

Hot Oil Fondue

2–4 cups avocado or extra virgin olive oil
4 ounces beef per person, cut in bite-sized cubes
2–4 ounces chicken breast per person, cut into thin strips
2 ounces per person medium size shrimp (cooked or
   uncooked), tails intact

Heat oil to 325–350F, either in the fondue pot if electric, which is best for oil, or on the stovetop for flame pots. If using a flame pot carefully transfer the hot oil to the fondue pot. Do not fill the pot more than 2/3 full, to reduce splashing over the rim of the pot while cooking. Pierce the raw meat or seafood with fondue forks and submerge in hot oil for about a minute. Remove and let cool briefly before dipping in sauce to eat.

Broth Fondue

4–6 cups chicken broth
2 tablespoons dry white wine*
1 garlic clove, thinly sliced
1 tablespoon fresh ginger, grated
3 tablespoons Worcestershire or gluten free soy sauce or coconut aminos
Salt and Pepper to taste
2–4 mushrooms per person, whole or halved, depending on size
4–6 broccoli crowns per person, blanched
2–4 cauliflower crowns per person, blanched
4–6 snow peas per person, blanched
2–3 mini carrots per person, blanched

Combine all ingredients (salt and pepper optional) into electric fondue pot or on a stovetop pot if using flame fondue pot. Bring liquid to a simmer (liquid is moving and steam coming off surface) and transfer to table for serving. Begin dipping.

For flame pots, bring liquid to a boil on the stove then carefully transfer to the flame fondue pot. Dip vegetables into broth until cooked to your liking, warm but still crisp, or soft and mushy. If you really want the vegetables cooked quickly, I recommend blanching all the vegetables (drop them for 2–5 minutes in boiling water, then stop the cooking process by dropping them in cold water, then drain) before cooking them in the broth. The blanching can be done in advance and then refrigerated until serving time.

*Alcohol can be replaced with broth, although the alcohol content will evaporate during the heating process, if there is a concern.

Chocolate Fondue

½ pound bittersweet chocolate (confirm the contents comply
with your eating style)
½ cup heavy cream or coconut milk
¼ teaspoon pure stevia powder (equivalent to 1/8 cup pure
cane or brown sugar)
2 tablespoons butter, avocado oil or coconut oil
2 teaspoons vanilla
Sweets and fruit cut into bite sized pieces, including
strawberries, bananas, melon, pineapple, mango,
marshmallows, pound or angel food cake.

Combine all ingredients in pot on stovetop or in a microwave-
proof glass bowl. Melt on low heat until liquid and well combined.
If using the microwave heat for 30 seconds and stir until mostly
melted, then stir until all lumps are gone. Whether prepared on the
stovetop or in the microwave, transfer to fondue pot for serving and
dip dip dip.

Lemon Ginger Sauce

Ginger sauce is a great marinade or dipping. If you have a hankering for Asian or any other ginger based flavor it is ideal. For fondue it is quintessential. Chicken likes it loads too!

Prep Time: 5 minutes

Cook Time: 10 minutes

Servings: 6

>½ cup coconut aminos (or gluten free soy/teriyaki sauce if you can tolerate soy)
>1 teaspoon fresh ground ginger (or ½ teaspoon ground ginger)
>3/8 teaspoon pure stevia powder (equivalent to ¼ cup pure cane sugar)
>2 tablespoons lemon juice
>Salt to taste

Add all ingredients to a pot on the stovetop. Heat until ingredients come to a gentle boil. Remove from heat and let cool. Salt to taste, for the coconut aminos may not be as salty as traditional soy sauce, so it may need help.

Serve as dipping sauce for chicken, fish or fondue. Store in an airtight container in the refrigerator.

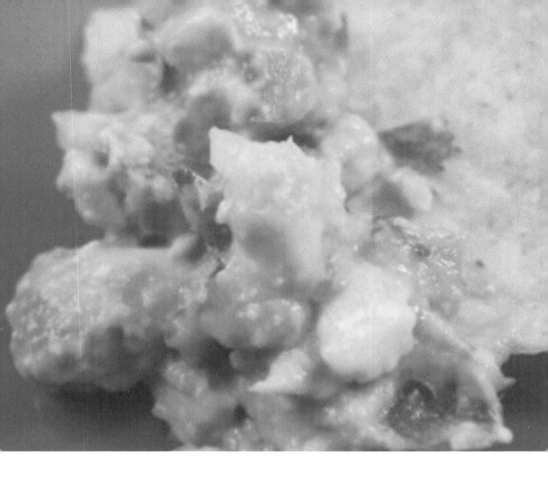

4 large ripe avocados
2 small tomatoes, diced with seeds removed
½ small white or red onion, diced
1 medium jalapeño, diced with seeds removed
  (or leave them in for spiciness)
1 lime, juiced and meat included
¼ cup fresh cilantro, roughly chopped
1 clove garlic, diced
½ teaspoon ground cumin
Salt and Pepper to taste

Guacamole

When I first started making guacamole at a teenager I would throw everything in a blender, add sour cream and make it a smooth, creamy dip. I don't recall why I started making it smooth, because I was surrounded by people who preferred creating chunky versions. Maybe it was my way of being a rebel–I toilet-papered a few houses and made smooth guacamole. Scary.

Now that I am a big girl I make it chunky. I really like not knowing if I am going to bite into a piece of tomato, onion, jalapeño or avocado. Here is how I do it.

Prep Time: 15 minutes

Cook Time: 1 hour for chilling

Servings: 32

Cut avocados in half lengthwise. Carefully remove the pit (I usually strike it with my knife blade and twist). In each half cut the avocado meat in a crisscross pattern. With a spoon scoop all the meat out of the skins into a medium bowl.

Add the remaining ingredients, keeping the lime juice for last to pour over the top. Stir it all together with a fork, adding salt and pepper to taste and smashing some of the avocado. To prevent the top from turning brown during storage, cover with cling wrap and press it down against the guacamole until all the air is pushed out. Chill for at least an hour before serving.

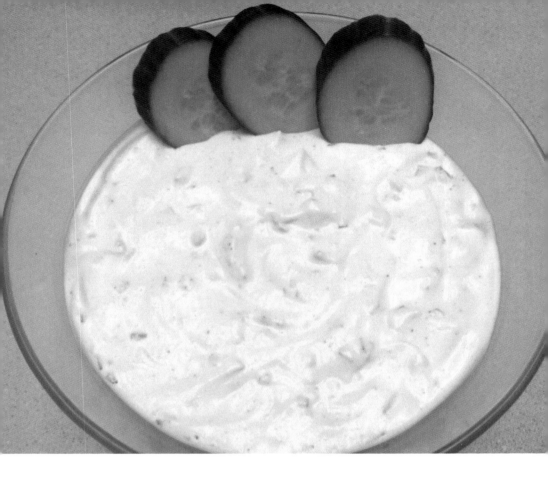

When joining a gathering of family and friends, there is always a need to nibble as people arrive and other foods are prepared. A healthy option is always veggies and dip, or more fancily called, crudite. Crudite is a traditional French appetizer consisting of sliced raw vegetables dipped in vinaigrette or dip. These three variations are great with veggies and any other dippable devices.

Variations on a Dip

Chive Goat Cheese Dip

The combination of the goat cheese, sour cream and mayonnaise made for a very tangy creamy dip base.

Prep Time: 10 minutes

Cook Time: 0

Servings: 40 heaping spoonfuls

> 1 cup goat cheese
> 1 cup sour cream
> ½ cup mayonnaise (in Sauces)
> 1 tablespoon lemon juice
> 1 handful fresh chives (about 1 cup chopped)
> ¼ cup finely chopped white onion
> 2 cloves finely chopped garlic
> 1 teaspoon salt

In a medium bowl, combine goat cheese, sour cream, and mayonnaise. Whisk until smooth. Add lemon juice, chives, onion, garlic and salt. Whisk more until everything is combined. Chill for at least an hour before serving.

Curry Dip

If you have a hankering for yellow curry but want something quick and cold, whip up this dip and have fun with it!

Prep Time: 5 minutes

Cook Time: 0

Servings: 16 heaping spoonfuls

1 cup unsweetened plain or greek yogurt
2 teaspoons ground turmeric
½ teaspoon ground black pepper
¼ teaspoon garlic powder
¼ teaspoon ground garlic
⅛ teaspoon ground ginger
1½ teaspoon lime juice
Salt and Pepper to taste

Mix all ingredients until well combined, including additional salt and black pepper to taste. Refrigerate until served.

Dill Dip

This dip is reminiscent of tzatziki and complements raw or steamed vegetables, and works well to coat baked meats as well, resulting in a complementary creamy sauce.

Prep Time: 10 minutes

Cook Time: 0

Servings: 24 heaping spoonfuls

1½ cups sour cream
1 fresh shallot, finely chopped
2 tablespoons fresh dill, finely chopped (use 1 tablespoon dried dill)
1 tablespoon lemon juice
Salt and Pepper to taste

Combine all ingredients well, including additional salt and black pepper to taste. Refrigerate until served.

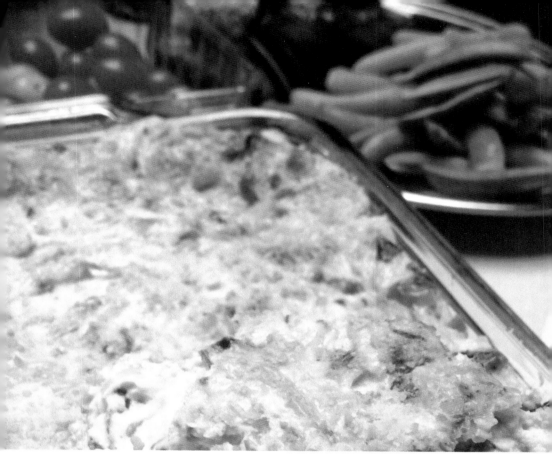

4 cups fresh spinach, roughly chopped
28 ounces (2 cans) artichoke hearts in water,
    drained and chopped
½ small yellow onion, finely chopped
32 ounces cream cheese, room temperature
1 cup sour cream
½ cup heavy cream
¼ cup Worcestershire sauce
4 garlic cloves, minced
½ bunch fresh parsley, finely chopped
2 tablespoons lemon juice
2 teaspoons salt
1 teaspoon ground black pepper
3 tablespoons grated Parmesan cheese

Spinach Artichoke Dip

The cool thing about this dip is that it freezes well so the volume will not go to waste. This is a big recipe! It can easily be halved for a smaller dose, but I like making it for parties and pot lucks, so I share below the big version.

Prep Time: 20 minutes

Cook Time: 45 minutes (plus 10 minutes cooling time)

Servings: 45 (¼ cup each)

Preheat oven to 350 degrees.

In a mixer bowl add all ingredients. Mix on medium speed for two minutes until all ingredients are thoroughly combined.

Pour mixture into 9x9 or larger baking dish and smooth top layer. Sprinkle Parmesan cheese on top.

Bake for 45 minutes until hot and bubbly. If top has not browned to your liking turn on the broiler and let broil until highest points turn brown. Watch closely to avoid burning.

Remove from oven and let rest for about ten minutes. Serve with vegetables or other dipping delicacies.

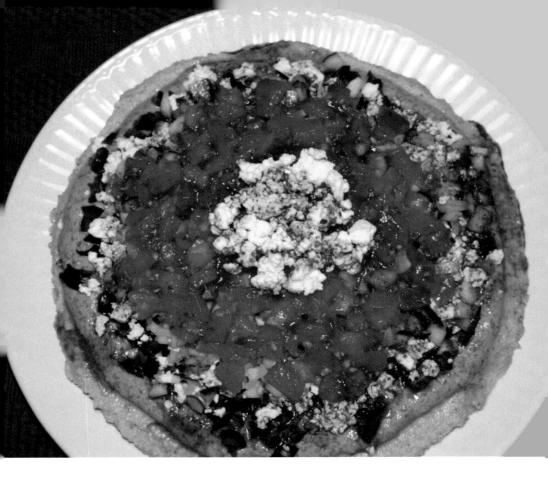

1 tablespoon olive oil
2 tablespoons balsamic vinegar
2 teaspoons chopped oregano
2 teaspoons lemon juice
Salt and Pepper to taste
2 cups prepared veggie hummus (See recipe in
  this Section)
1 cup plain Greek yogurt (optional)*
2-3 cups raw spinach
1 cup feta cheese, crumbled
1 cup cucumber, chopped
1 large tomato, chopped
1 cup kalamata olives, chopped

Greek Layer Dip

Sometimes when a big gaggle of people are coming over I like making available a variety of appetizers so they can nibble as they trickle into the house. One of my favorites is a layer dip. It is high in fiber and very colorful. It can also substitute for a green salad if you have enough Greek lovers.

It is nice if you have a robust vegetable garden, for this dip is a great way to use up some of the bumper crops for friend and neighbors later this year.

Prep Time: 20 minutes

Cook Time: 0

Servings: 28 (¼ cup each)

Combine in small bowl the oil, vinegar, oregano, salt, pepper and lemon juice. Set aside. Spread hummus on a serving tray in an even layer, about ¼ to ½ inch deep. Chop spinach into small pieces (and if you are using yogurt now is the time to combine the yogurt with spinach until well blended)*.

Spread/sprinkle the spinach on top of the hummus, leaving a visible edge of hummus. Sprinkle olives on top of spinach mixture, followed by cucumber and tomato. Drizzle dressing on top of dip and add some more feta for garnish if you like, then serve. It can be prepared about two hours in advance and chilled until serving.

*If you are making the dip more than two hours in advance, I would recommend the yogurt not be used. Depending on the brand of yogurt, it can be a runny layer and will spread. It should hold up if made within an hour or two of serving. I have made it both with the yogurt and without–just sprinkling a layer of spinach makes it look different, but still beautiful and you will still have a moist, dippable dip.

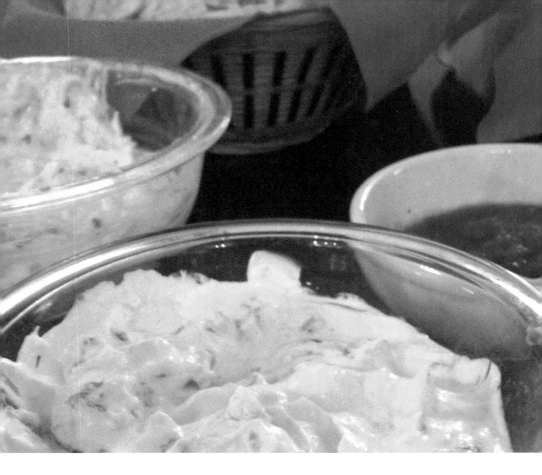

2 cups sour cream
1 tablespoon lime juice
1 tablespoon ground cumin
1 teaspoon garlic powder
1 teaspoon salt
½ teaspoon ground black pepper
1 can (14.5 ounces) tomato and chiles, well
  drained
¼ cup finely chopped onion

Tex Mex Dip

Dip is a sure-fire thing to always have around. Having last minute dinner guests? Pull out the dip with crudite. Feeling nibbly? Pull out the dip with some pork rinds. Faced with raw chicken that needs to be dinner? Pull out the dip and slather the fowl with it before tossing it in the oven.

Headed over to someone's place for drinks? Pull out the dip, put it in a fancy bowl and take it along with you. It can come in all shapes and sizes and colors and quantities. It can be hot, or cold or both. People can eat it, or not. Dips can be made to taste like just about any dish.

We like queso. When we don't want to break out the crock pot or deal with hot food we don't have to miss out on the flavors. We just pull out the can of chiles and tomatoes and veer in another direction.

Prep Time: 8 minutes

Cook Time: 0

Servings: 12 (¼ cup each)

In a medium bowl combine sour cream, lime juice, cumin, garlic, salt and pepper. Whisk until combined. Add onion, tomatoes and chiles. Stir until well combined. Chill at least two hours or overnight before serving.

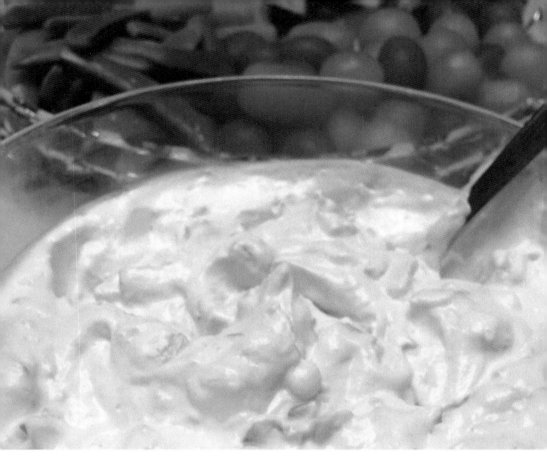

1 large or two small onion (Vidalia works great for sweeter
   result, but any yellow or white type will do)
2 cups water
1 cup sour cream or plain Greek yogurt
1 cup mayonnaise (see Sauces section for recipe)
2 cloves garlic, minced
2 tablespoon dijon mustard
1 teaspoon celery salt
Salt and Pepper to taste

French Onion Dip

My favorite dip EVER is French onion dip. Onion soup has been around since recorded ancient Roman times, but French onion soup was the inspiration for the dip which became popular in the United States about 60 years ago. I have not asked any of them lately, but I bet the French would happily disown the dip version of their lovely soup.

Growing up, we always had packets of French onion soup mix in the pantry. I was in my 30s before I actually used the mix to make soup. Until then I had only used the packets for making dip or seasoning meats.

I have since been looking closely at ingredients of everything I buy, especially anything processed or convenient. Yup. Convenience is extremely suspicious to me these days. This close looking led me to the back of the French onion soup mix: sugar, corn syrup, monosodium glutamate…I am pretty sure the Romans did not use much of those in their onion soup, and I am not keen on consuming them. It is easy to make packet-free French onion dip, and it is fun too! It takes a bit longer, but if you are in the kitchen doing other things anyway, you probably won't notice.

Have you ever caramelized onions? It is a kitchen task I always enjoy if I have the time. Onion, water and a little salt makes for impressive results. The biggest challenge is carefully watching while they cook (but not burn) and avoiding the temptation to stir.

Prep Time: 10 minutes

Cook Time: 25 minutes (plus 2 hours chilling time)

Servings: 12 (¼ cup each)

Roughly chop the onion, making sure all the pieces are broken up. Heat a medium saute pan to medium high heat. When the pan is hot add the onion to the dry pan. Let cook for about five minutes without stirring, allowing the onion to release moisture and begin to brown. Toss onion and let cook undisturbed for another three minutes.

Add ½ cup water and stir, making sure to scrape the brown bits from the bottom of the pan. Let cook undisturbed for another 3 - 5 minutes, allowing the liquid to reduce. When liquid is almost gone and onions begin to brown and caramelize again, stir and add another ½ cup of water. Repeat the liquid reduction and stirring two more times, until all the water is incorporated.*

Sprinkle onions with ¼ teaspoon salt. Stir and set aside to cool. In a medium bowl combine the sour cream, mayonnaise, garlic, mustard, celery salt, pepper and more salt to taste. Add the cooled onions and stir until combined.

Refrigerate at least two hours or overnight before serving. Serve with vegetables, chips and crackers.

*The caramelized onions can also be made in advance and pureed, to be used for a variety of recipes that call for onion, including this dip, if you prefer a quicker preparation.

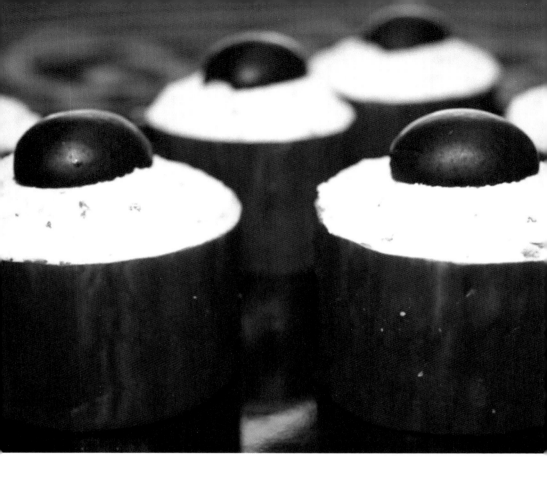

1 English cucumber, washed, peel on
5 ounces goat cheese, room temperature
1 teaspoon dried parsley leaves
½ teaspoon dried basil leaves
½ teaspoon garlic powder
8-10 extra large black olives, drained and patted
  dry
Salt and Pepper to taste

Cucumber Goat Cheese Bites

I think my first experience eating goat cheese was in Golden, Colorado, while lunching in a little cafe in the historic downtown area. It was spread on a chicken sandwich, in lieu of mustard or other condiments. I remember leaning on the table with my eyes closed, wondering where the cheese had been all my life.

Granted, I was only 25 or so, but it seemed such a long time to have been without goat cheese! Since that first, fateful chicken sandwich I scour menus for it and grab packages now and then from the store. I get unreasonably excited when a restaurant offers a dollop on top of an otherwise basic green salad, or includes it in a cheesy dippy appetizer.

Here is a simple cold appetizer, or green salad substitute, that combines flavors my family and I love.

Prep Time: 15 minutes

Cook Time: 0

Servings: 8-10

Cut cucumber into ⅓ to ½ inch long slices. Scoop out an indentation about ¼ inch deep on one end of each slice, which will be filled with a cheese mixture. You can use a small melon baller or ½ teaspoon size scoop.

Stir together cheese, parsley, basil and garlic. Sprinkle indentations and tops of cucumber slices with salt and pepper.

Using a spoon place some goat cheese mixture on top of each slice, filling the indentation and creating a smooth mound rising up about ¼ inch above the top of the cucumber.

Slice olives in half lengthwise, then place a half on top of each cucumber slice.

Chill until served.

DRESSINGS
&
SAUCES

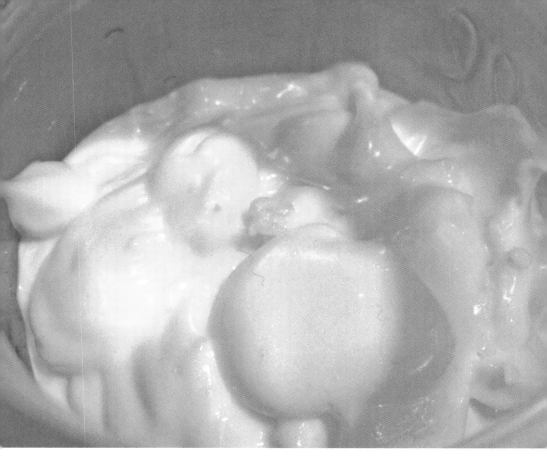

1 egg yolk
1 egg
1 cup avocado oil
2 tablespoons lemon juice
¼–½ teaspoon salt

Mayonnaise

Since I was a kid I always liked the taste of mayonnaise; the smooth creaminess it gave to sandwiches, sauces and recipes. I fondly remember lunching on many ham and cheese sandwiches layered with tomatoes, pickles and a nice combination of mayo and mustard mixed up with it all.

The sandwiches, along with the occasional dollop on a tomato or tossing it in tuna salad, bring back memories of hot summer days, and loud lunches in school cafeterias.

I am particular about my mayonnaise. I like it tart and creamy. Our first forays into making mayonnaise tasted good but were not quite a replacement for the flavor of my youth. You might not be as picky about the taste as I am, but we tried this version recently and it hit the mark! We are pretty sure it is the avocado oil that took it over the edge as a true substitute for my beloved mayo.

Olive oil works well, too, but the flavor of olive oil takes it in a different direction. This is such an easy recipe that works every time and keeps me away from the store stuff, which is soy-filled, sugar-filled and preserved with the nasty calcium disodium EDTA.

This mayonnaise can be used in lieu of the store bought mayonnaise, as well as cream or milk in savory sauces. We use it as a base for our Ranch Dressing too!

Prep Time: 5 minutes

Cook Time: 0

Servings: 16 tablespoons

Place egg yolk and egg in a blender, turning it on medium speed.

Slowly add oil to the eggs in a narrow, steady stream until fully incorporated.

Add lemon juice while the mixture continues to blend. Stir in salt to desired taste.

Remove mayonnaise to a glass container that can be sealed air-tight. Store in refrigerator.

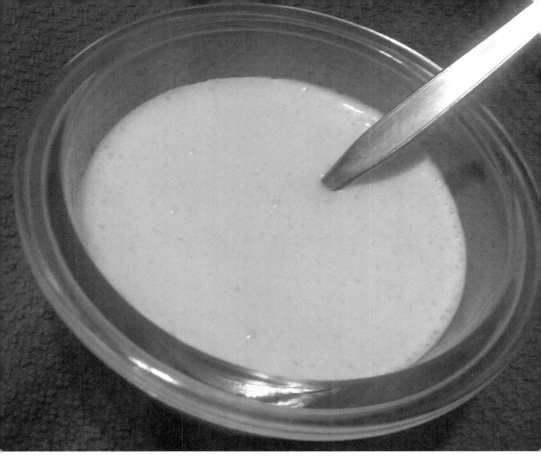

4 ounces butter
2 egg yolks
1 tablespoon lemon juice or vinegar
1 tablespoon water
¼ teaspoon salt (you may need less if
  using salted butter)

Hollandaise Sauce

Hollandaise sauce is one of the five French mother sauces, made for hundreds of years to enhance egg, vegetable and meat dishes around the world. As a mother sauce, it can be used to make other classic variations by adding a few simple ingredients.

Prep Time: 8 minutes

Cook Time: 0

Servings: 4

Melt the butter and let cool briefly. While butter is cooling add the rest of ingredients in a blender but do not blend them yet. When butter has cooled a bit spoon out the foamy, bubbly top from butter, leaving the clear, yellow clarified portion.

Use only the clarified portion for the sauce. Begin blending the mixed ingredients on low and gradually and steadily add the butter. Let blend for about a minute. Stop the blender. Leave sauce at room temperature until served.

This recipe can be multiplied as needed, without adjusting any quantities.

After making the base sauce, the following ingredients can be added to make other traditional sauces. They can be used on fish, meat, or vegetables that are otherwise complemented by the noted additions.

Sauce Choron: add a teaspoon of tomato sauce.
Sauce Bavaroise: add ¼ teaspoon of horseradish and pinch of thyme.
Sauce Crème Fleurette: add a tablespoon of sour cream.
Sauce Dijon: add a teaspoon of dijon or other sharp mustard.
Sauce Maltaise: add ½ teaspoon of orange zest and a tablespoon of orange juice.
Sauce Mousseline: add 2 tablespoons of whipped cream.
Sauce Noisette: replace clarified butter with browned butter.

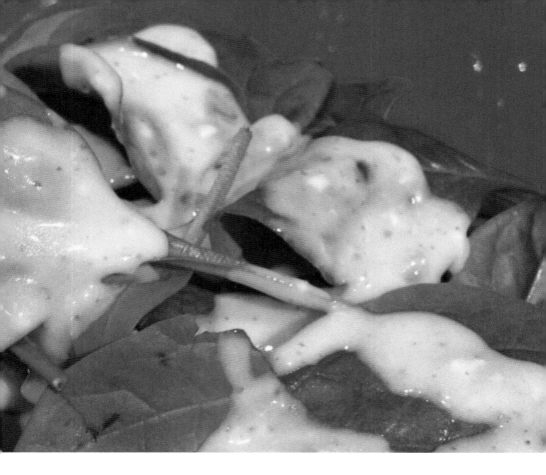

4 slices bacon

¼ cup water

¼ cup Apple cider vinegar

1/16 teaspoon pure stevia powder (equivalent to 1 tablespoon pure cane sugar)

1 tablespoon horseradish mustard (or 2 teaspoon yellow mustard and 1 teaspoon raw grated horseradish)

1 egg

Pinch salt (Optional)

¼ red onion, jullienne (Optional)

4 soft boiled eggs (6 minute boiled or 2 minute Instant Pot quick release)

Hot Bacon Dressing

The term "hot" as used for this recipe can mean two things—spicy hot and temperature hot. Other versions of the dressing can be heated up much more so as to clearly wilt the spinach as it is poured. This version, since it relies on egg as a thickener instead of flour or other powders, cannot be made so hot without curdling the egg.

I rely on the spicy version of the word "hot" here instead. The tang of the vinegar, along with the heat of the horseradish and mustard, make it so. It will probably not wilt the spinach, but it will still leave a mark on your palate. Besides serving it over spinach the dressing can also go on top of other side dishes, for it has a tang that would complement broccoli, squash, asparagus, and more.

If you heat up leftover dressing do it gradually in the microwave at half power or low on the stove so as not to create scrambled eggs.

Prep Time: 5 minutes

Cook Time: 10 minutes

Servings: 10 tablespoons

Cook the bacon over medium high heat in small pan until crisp. Crumble bacon and set aside. Turn temperature to low under bacon grease and let cool to the lower temperature. Add water, vinegar, sweetener and mustard, stirring until combined.

Whisk in egg and continue stirring constantly so the egg does not cook firm. When the egg is fully incorporated, add crumbled bacon, continuing to cook and stir under heated through. Taste and add salt if needed. Turn heat up to medium, continuing to stir, and heat until steam rises from the dressing, about two minutes.

Serve immediately over raw baby spinach, optionally including onion slices or soft boiled eggs sliced in half.

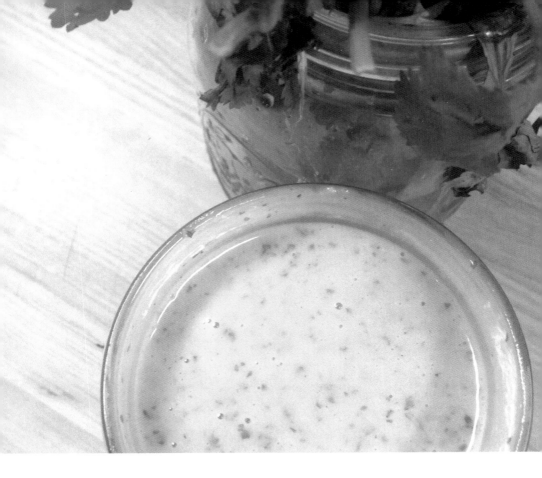

1 cup chopped fresh cilantro leaves
¼ cup fresh parsley leaves
⅛ cup fresh oregano leaves
⅔ cup apple cider vinegar
1 lime, juiced
½ cup extra virgin olive oil
2 garlic cloves, crushed
1 teaspoon salt
¼ teaspoon ground black pepper

Herby Dressing

After being surrounded by herbs one summer I decided to try and capture it all in a jar. I trundled through the jungle of herbs in the back yard and grabbed handfuls of garlic, cilantro and parsley. We use it so far to flavor salad, cottage cheese and dip. The word "dressing" may be deceiving, for it is not just for salad. It can brighten up all kinds of foods, so go for it!

Prep Time: 15 minutes

Cook Time: 0

Servings: 16 (2 tablespoons each)

Place all ingredients except for olive oil into a food processor. Pulse the ingredients until herbs are of a uniform size. Continue processing steadily while incorporating oil with a continuous, steady stream into the processor.

Store dressing in an airtight container, drizzling it with abandon on salads or incorporating it into meat dishes as a marinade.

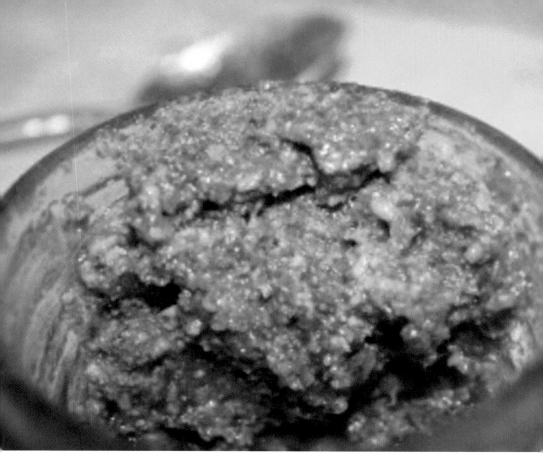

1 bunch fresh cilantro, most thicker stems
   removed
¼ - ⅓ cup extra virgin olive oil
4 cloves garlic
¼ cup pecan halves
¼ cup grated Parmesan cheese
½ jalapeño, seeds removed
½ teaspoon salt
1 tablespoon lime Juice

Cilantro Pesto

In Texas, cilantro is a spring crop. As the heat of summer arrives the plants start to fade. Here is what we do with the abundant harvest as we race to fully utilize the plants. It freezes well so if you are in over your head with cilantro you now have a way of redeeming yourself as an herb grower!

Prep Time: 20 minutes

Cook Time: 0

Servings: 16 tablespoons

Add all ingredients except oil to blender or food processor. Purée until blended, then slowly drizzle oil into mixture. Scrape sides and blend more until everything is about the same size.
Use immediately or chill until about an hour before serving. Room temperature is the best for serving. Additional volume can be frozen and thawed slowly in the refrigerator - it will be darker but still taste lovely.

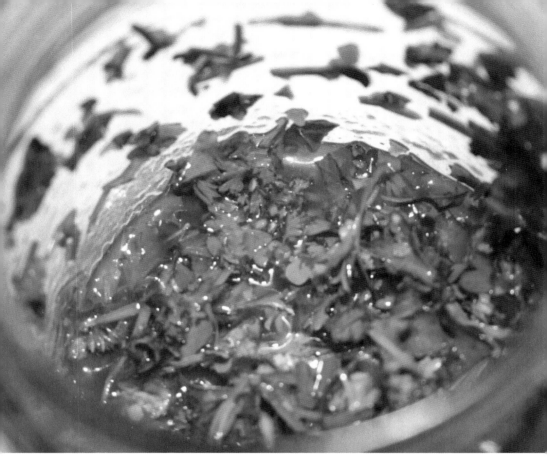

1 bunch parsley
1 clove garlic, crushed
1 teaspoon salt
1 lime, juiced with meat included
1 slice bacon, cooked crisp
1 tablespoon bacon grease
½ - ¾ cup olive oil or avocado oil

Chimichurri

I was first introduced to chimichurri in a restaurant in San Antonio. Drizzle a little on a chip or pork rind and crunch away! I don't know why, but I always want to eat more. I would not have thought a sauce made primarily of parsley would appease my palate, but it does. Besides the digestive benefits of the parsley, if made correctly the sauce has a gentle balance of tangy, soft and addictive.

It also goes wonderfully with pretty much any grilled meat, and of course drizzled over a fajita taco.

I have even used the final dredges of a jar to sear veggies. It can be made without the bacon and grease for a vegetarian version, but be warned the texture and depth changes. Make the chimichurri, and refrigerate it the day before you plan on serving it, and the flavors really meld together. You can actually make it the same day, but sitting overnight makes a noticeable difference.

Prep Time: 20 minutes

Cook Time: 0 (plus chilling the day before use)

Servings: 32 tablespoons

Chop parsley roughly, including stems (If chopped too small the leaves can taste bitter). Place them in a glass bowl or jar. Add garlic, salt, lime and oil. Stir or shake up the ingredients until the parsley is coated.

Heat up the bacon grease and chopped bacon until it is hot, then drizzle it over the mixture—this step will wilt some of the parsley and release flavor and aroma.

If you make the sauce the day before, you may want to pull it out of the fridge an hour or so before mealtime so it can warm to room temperature, because sometimes the fats will solidify when cold. Serve over meats or vegetables, or use as a dipping sauce.

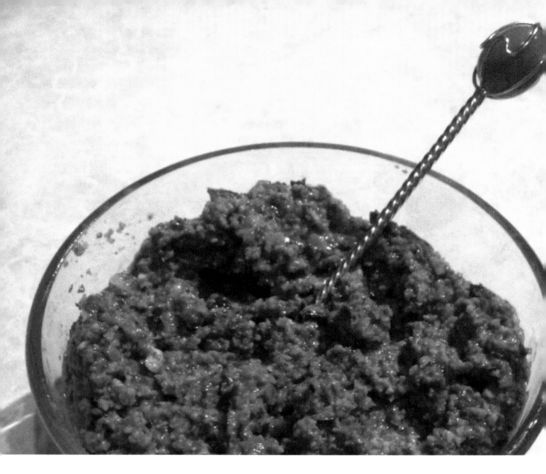

2 cups mixed black and green olives, pitted
3 cloves garlic
¼ cup small capers
¼ cup extra virgin olive oil
1 teaspoon dried oregano leaves
1 teaspoon dried basil leaves
1 teaspoon dried parsley leaves
1 anchovy fillet (optional)

Olive Tapenade

My early New Orleans connection is via lovely sandwiches that first introduced me to tapenade when I was a kid. Muffuletta sandwiches are about as common in New Orleans as po'boy sandwiches and gumbo. They originated in the Central Grocery right there on Decatur Street in the French Quarter.

When I first had one, I could not get enough of the olive "salad" in the sandwich. Between the olives and the meats and cheeses it was a very satisfying meal. To do a version of the sandwich that fits our eating habits, I make up some low carb bread, whipped up a batch of tapenade in the food processor, and opened up a few packages of deli meats and cheeses.

Any tapenade leftovers you may have need not go to waste—I have used it as a dip, or as a stuffing for chicken, pork and mushrooms. It has an addictive saltiness that, believe it or not, sates the salty snacking craving I used to appease by eating chips. Just a straight spoonful can do the trick!

Prep Time: 20 minutes

Cook Time: 0

Servings: 24 tablespoons

Place all ingredients, except the olive oil, into a food processor*. Slowly add the olive oil in a stream while the mixture is blending on low speed, until the mixture is an evenly sized paste. Serve as condiment for sandwiches, or with crackers as a dip. Store refrigerated in an air-tight container.

*If you want a chunkier tapenade, skip the food processor and manually chop all the ingredients until evenly sized. Stir the mixture briskly with a whisk while slowly adding the olive oil.

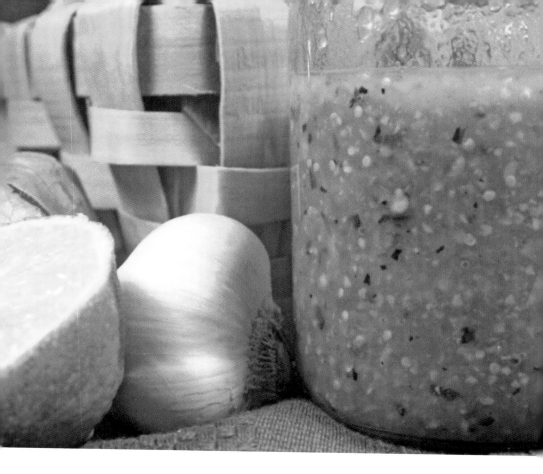

1 pound fresh tomatillos
1 small yellow onion
1 - 3 jalapenos (depending on desired spiciness)
1 garlic clove, crushed
1 lime, juiced with meat
¼ cup chopped cilantro
Pinch of pure stevia (optional)
Salt to taste (optional)

*I know the urge will be strong to take the pan out before the skins are truly black and smoking, but it really expands the flavor of the results if you control yourself and let them go black!

Salsa Verde With Tomatillos

I did not really get much salsa verde until I started traveling to New Mexico about ten years ago. Each restaurant served the sauce with varying levels of heat, from mild and sweet and almost dessert-like all the way to an addictive spiciness that leads to consuming many a chip and drinking margaritas much too fast.

Further south and west, the sauce is usually heavier on the peppers than my version, but I dug into my Tex-Mex roots for this recipe and used only one jalapeno. Since jalapeno heat varies, it is important to judge the number of peppers (and seeds, as described below) to include. If the tomatillos are nice and tangy and the onion a bit sweet, you may needed no sugar or salt at all.

Prep Time: 30 minutes

Cook Time: 30 minutes (plus at least 1 hour chilling)

Servings: 24 (¼ cup each)

Remove husks from tomatillos, wash well and cut in half. Remove dry layers from onion and cut it in half. Cut jalapeno in half. Remove seeds and discard if you want a milder salsa.

Set oven to high broil. Place tomatillos, jalapenos and onion on a broiling pan covered in aluminum foil, skin side up. The onion and jalapeno pieces should be on the outer edges, with the tomatillos in the center. Place under broiler and roast until tomatillo skins begin to blacken/char, at least 5 minutes and possibly up to 10, depending on the power of your broiler. Rotate the pan and broil longer if needed to maximize blackening*. Remove from oven and let vegetables cool.

Combine all ingredients, except stevia and salt, in a food processor and pulse to desired texture, or use a molcajete and break it up the old fashioned way.

Place salsa in a pot on the stove over medium heat covered. When it is hot turn it down to continue simmering for 30 minutes. Remove from heat and let cool. Place in airtight container.

Refrigerate for at least an hour, but ideally overnight. Add stevia and/or salt to taste if needed before serving. The flavor of the tomatillos and char can vary, so I recommend waiting until the next day to adjust the flavor.

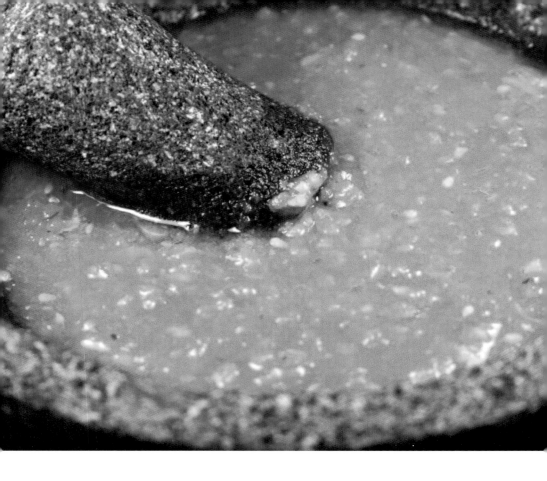

4 large rip tomatoes, quartered
½ small red onion, roughly chopped
1 large or 2 small jalapenos (more if
  stronger heat desired), roughly chopped
1 lime, juiced with meat included
3 cloves garlic
¼ teaspoon ground cumin
1 small bunch cilantro
½ teaspoon ground salt

Tomato Salsa

Salsa! It is low fat, low calorie, low sugar, and can spice up pretty much anything. I have made it cold, warm, roasted, raw, green, brown (it was actually good) and, of course, red. The raw red version is the one that most reminds me of the tex-mex restaurants I like the most down in Texas where I grew up.

Each batch turns out a little different, depending on the quality of the tomatoes and the bite of the jalapenos. This version of salsa comes straight out of the fridge. It is raw, red and tangy. I made the recipe mild, but it could of course be spiced up with more jalapenos.

Prep Time: 15 minutes

Cook Time: 0 (plus chill overnight)

Servings: 22 (¼ cup each)

If you have a big food processor, combine one tomato with the remaining ingredients and pulse until finely pureed. Add remaining tomatoes and pulse until roughly chopped. Refrigerate overnight and serve cold.

If you are going to use a molcajete, combine the onion, jalapeno, lime meat, garlic and cilantro in a bowl. Grind until all the ingredients are combined. Add tomatoes and continue grinding until combined and the tomatoes are of your preferred mushiness. Refrigerate overnight and serve cold.

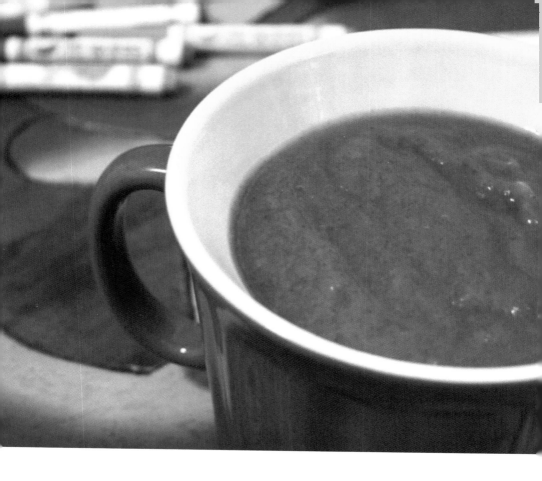

6–8 large Granny Smith apples
1 tablespoon ground cinnamon
1 cup water

Tart Apple Sauce

If your local grocer is anything like mine, they have a corner of the produce section where you can occasionally find deeply discounted apples that are gently bruised. Making apple sauce with them results in a nice, tart result. I think it tastes much better than the sweeter stuff from the store. I don't add any sweetener or sugar—I don't think the sauce, or our family, needs it, but sweetener could easily be added if you prefer.

Prep Time: 10 minutes

Cook Time: 30 minutes - 6 hours depending on cooking method

Servings: 8 (½ cup each)

Core and slice apples, leaving the skin on. The skin will soften and cook down, so you won't notice it in the final product. The sauce will be darker than what you typically buy at the store, but the texture is the same.

Place apples in a crock pot. Add cinnamon and toss to coat the apple slices. Pour water over apples, cover and set temperature to low. Cook for 6–8 hours*. Let cool and puree with a hand mixer or food processor until smooth. Store in the refrigerator or freezer.

*If you want quicker results, cook covered in a medium sized pot on low for about two hours. Another option is using a pressure cooker for 10 minutes with natural release.

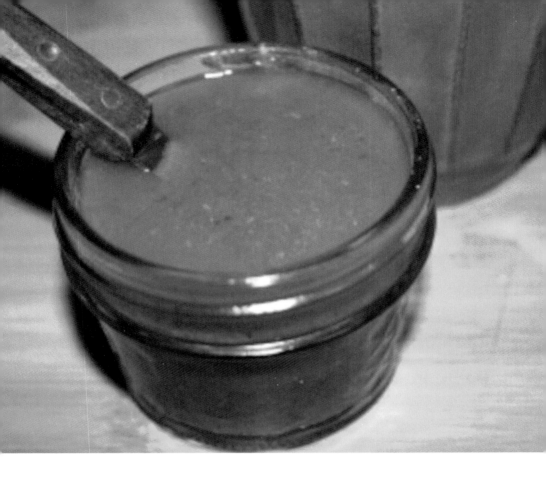

1 cup water
1½ teaspoons pure stevia powder (equivalent to 1 cup pure cane sugar)
⅓ cup pureed pumpkin
1 teaspoon ground cinnamon
½ inch fresh ginger finely grated, or 1 teaspoon ground ginger
½ teaspoon ground nutmeg
¼ teaspoon ground clove
1 teaspoon vanilla extract

Pumpkin Spice Syrup

Oh my! The taste of Autumn! For winter, I want peppermint and eggnog. Spring reminds me of berries and fresh salads. Summer is the chill of popsicles and fresh produce everywhere. Now, Autumn. Autumn is squash and cinnamon, nutmeg and clove–and this syrup is the quintessence of fall.

I enjoy the chill in the air, along with hot teas and coffees. One of my favorite indulgences is the pumpkin spice lattes popping up in coffee shops everywhere. The problem is all the sugar in them and the expense, which are discouraging elements.

This sugar free syrup has just the right mix of sweet and spicy, without spiking blood sugar. It can also be drizzled over ice cream, stirred into hot tea, or mixed with hot chocolate as well. You won't be able to get enough. Yum!

Prep Time: 5 minutes

Cook Time: 15 minutes plus cooling time

Servings: 24 tablespoons

Combine pumpkin, water and stevia in medium sauce pan. Cook over medium heat until everything is dissolved and begins to bubble.

Add cinnamon, ginger, nutmeg, clove and vanilla. Simmer on low, stirring frequently, for about ten minutes until the syrup thickens and makes the house smell wonderful. Let cool to room temperature.

At this point you can do one of two things: Option 1) store in glass jar in the fridge, or Option 2) strain through fine sieve into a glass jar and store it in the fridge. If you don't mind stirring your coffee while you drink it, don't worry about straining and do option one.

If you want a more blended cup of coffee or aim to use the syrup in a latte, then do option two. If used in a latte, add about one tablespoon for every cup of milk. The syrup also goes well drizzled over ice cream, warm muffins, cinnamon rolls, or stirred in with pancake syrup for an autumn twist.

BREAKFASTS

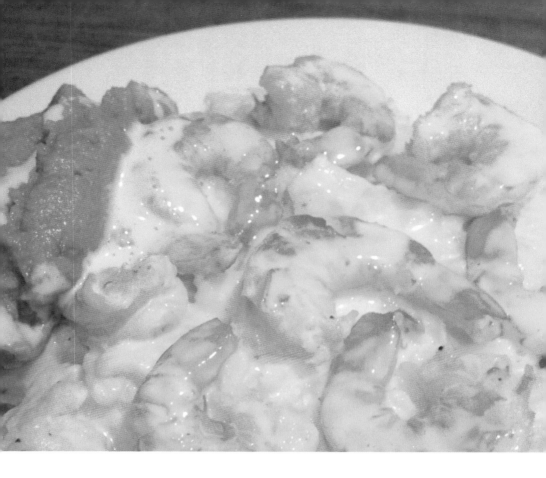

12 eggs*
¼ teaspoon salt
Dash of ground black pepper
1 tablespoon butter
½ pound medium shrimp, deveined, shells and tails
   removed*
½ lemon
1 teaspoon salt
1 avocado, peeled and sliced
Hollandaise sauce (see recipe in Sauces)

*The egg, shrimp, and sauce quantities assume six servings. You can always make fewer servings and have sauce left over if it is a better fit for your meal plans.

Shrimp Hollandaise On Eggs

We eat a lot of eggs. Not only are they good sources of protein, they are extremely versatile. Do you want to bake some cookies? Add an egg. Do you want to thicken a casserole? Add an egg. Do you want a shiny finish on your pie crust? Brush it with an egg wash. Do you want a fun appetizer or side dish? Devil some. Need to feed a crowd of overnight guests? Make a frittata. Do you want a breakfast that sticks to your ribs? Scramble some.

You can always throw some meat and cheese into your scrambled egg, but there is that occasional morning when you want something different.

Here is a dish for one of those different days. My original craving was for Eggs Benedict, but I have not yet mastered the grain free English muffin, so I deviated. I figured out that what I was craving was the Hollandaise Sauce. Although not a traditional, more complicated version of the sauce, this was quick to make and ready in advance of the short cooking time needed for the shrimp and eggs.

Prep Time: 20 minutes

Cook Time: 20 minutes

Servings: 6

Fill a medium pot half with water. Add salt, squeeze lemon juice into water and drop the lemon half into the water. Set pot over high heat. While waiting for water to boil for the shrimp, make Hollandaise Sauce.

When water is boiling, add shrimp, cover and turn off heat. Let sit for no more than three minutes, just until they turn pink all over. Remove from water and place on towel to drain.

In a bowl, crack the eggs and add salt and pepper. Whisk until combined.

In a frying pan, melt butter over medium high heat. Add eggs and stir in the pan until cooked to desired doneness. Divide eggs among individual serving plates. Top with shrimp, then drizzle them with Hollandaise sauce.

Add avocado slices or guacamole and serve.

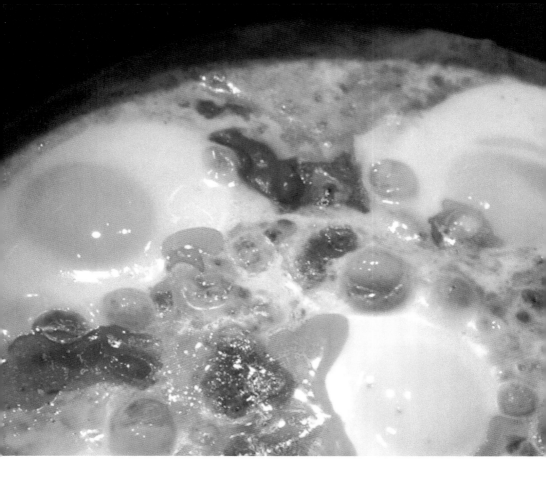

2 tablespoons butter or oil
½ white onion, finely chopped
4 cloves garlic, finely chopped
½ cup natural peanut butter
15 ounces tomato sauce
½ cup lemon juice
2 tablespoons ground turmeric
2 teaspoons ground ginger
1 teaspoon ground cinnamon
1 tablespoon cayenne pepper
1 teaspoon salt
1 teaspoon ground black pepper
8 ounces full fat coconut milk
3 - 6 eggs

Red Eggs

This anytime-of-day egg dish is reminiscent of Indian shakshuka or Mexican huevos rancheros, and the concept sounded really good, easy and filling. The sauce is reminiscent of Indian Butter Chicken, which I absolutely love. It can also be dairy free if you substitute oil for the butter. Beware and do not step away from the pan at the wrong minute, ensuring the poachiness of the eggs is what you want.

Prep Time: 10 minutes

Cook Time: 25 minutes

Servings: 3

In a medium saute pan over medium high heat, melt butter or oil. Add the onion and garlic, cooking until browning begins, about five minutes.

Add the remaining ingredients, except for coconut milk. Stir until all ingredients are combined, turning down heat to low. Stir in coconut milk and simmer until steam is rising from sauce, about ten minutes.

With the back of a spoon, make a divot along the edge of the sauce in the pan. Drop a raw egg into the divet. Repeat with the remaining eggs, evenly distributing them in the sauce.

Cover pan and let simmer until eggs are cooked to desired doneness—about five minutes for soft.

Serve immediately by scooping egg(s) onto a plate and drizzle sauce on top. If there is extra sauce, it can be refrigerated in an air-tight container and used another time.

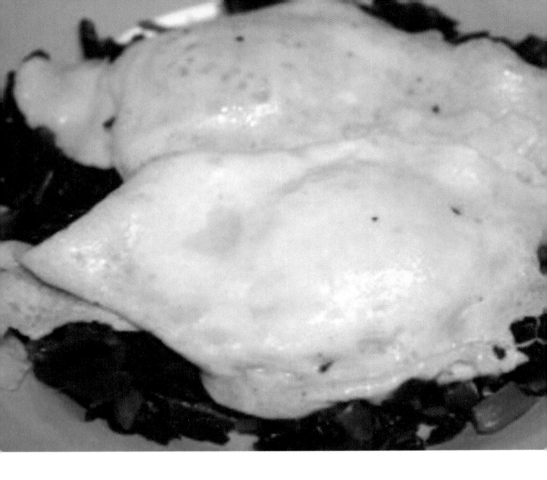

3 tablespoons butter, salted
2 cloves garlic, crushed
4 cups frozen collard greens and/or
  spinach, chopped
4–6 eggs
Salt and pepper to taste

Eggs And Greens

The combination of protein and fiber in this dish will fill up your tummy, and doesn't take very long to throw together. We like keeping greens in the freezer that were previously blanched, so a quick saute will make instant, hot veggies for us. We always, always have eggs around, so the combination is a no brainer.

The recipe as written should result in eggs cooked medium. Medium makes for some firm parts to munch with the egg whites, while the runny part mix up with the greens. More or less time is needed if you prefer other than medium eggs.

Prep Time: 5 minutes

Cook Time: 15 minutes

Servings: 3

In a sauté pan over medium high heat, add 1 tablespoon butter. When butter is melted, add garlic and toss until garlic sweats. Add greens and toss until wilted and heated through, about five minutes. Sprinkle with salt and pepper to taste and toss. Remove from heat, cover and set aside. The greens will continue to soften and keep warm, but not lose much more in the way of nutritional benefit.

In a medium sauté pan, add 2 tablespoons butter over medium heat. When butter is melted, crack all four eggs into the pan. Gently push the edges of the eggs towards the yolks so the pan doesn't become one big four-eyed egg. Sprinkle with just a bit of salt.

After just enough time to let the eggs set, turn down the heat to low. You can either:

1) flip each egg separately and cook for another minute, or

2) if you don't like flipping, just cover the pan for a minute, allowing the top of the eggs to set.

Either way, nudge the yolks gently to monitor the speed of cooking, until they are cooked to desired doneness–soft, medium or hard. To plate, divide the greens among 2-4 plates, then flatten them a bit. Add one to two eggs on top of each. Serve immediately.

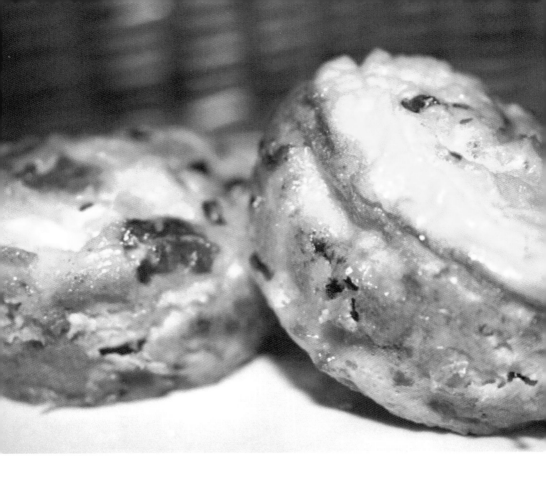

2 cups eggs
1 cup frozen spinach
1 cup cheese, grated
½ cup ham or cooked sausage, small dice
¼ cup black olives, chopped
Salt and pepper to taste
2 teaspoons dried parsley
½ teaspoon garlic powder
¼ teaspoon onion powder

Eggy Muffins

When my stomach is grumbling first thing in the morning, it is almost torture waiting for yummy bits to cook that accompany eggs–the bacon or potatoes to crisp, the sausage patties to sear, the making of Hollandaise sauce or the baking of buns.

My favorite solution is baking little quiche-like 'muffins'–they can be eaten immediately, or pulled from the fridge or freezer and heated up later, while retaining their savory goodness. The content of each batch of muffins I make varies and is directly impacted by the content of my kitchen. They always have eggs and cheese, but the meat and veggies change constantly–leftover roast chicken and broccoli are popular additions, as are grilled pork chops and greens. Muffins with salmon, dill and asparagus are wonderful.

Prep Time: 30 minutes

Cook Time: 25 minutes

Servings: 12

Heat oven to 375F. Grease a 12-count muffin pan. In the microwave, cook the spinach for about two minutes in a covered dish. While it cools, prepare the rest of the dish.

In a medium-sized bowl add the cheese, meats and olives. Stir together.

Crack all eggs into a separate bowl. Add salt, pepper, garlic, onion powder and parsley. Whisk the eggs until whites and yolks are well blended.

When spinach is cool enough to handle, squeeze as much liquid out as possible. Chop finely and add to meat/veggie mixture. Stir until spinach is well incorporated.

Spoon mixture into muffin pan until it is evenly distributed among the 12 spaces.

Pour the egg mixture over the cheese, meats and vegetables in the muffin pan. Each divot should be 2/3 to 3/4 full. Gently stir everything together to make sure some of the egg settles in the bottom of the divot.

Bake in preheated oven for 15-20 minutes until they start to brown on top. Remove from oven and let muffins cool in pan for about five minutes. Run a knife around the edge of each round to separate them from the pan, then gently lift them out onto a serving dish. Serve immediately or freeze.

To reheat frozen muffins, microwave for 20 seconds, adding five seconds for each additional muffin heated simultaneously.

NOTE: If you change around the kinds of proteins, vegetables or cheeses, just make sure the egg/cheese/filling ratios stay consistent, otherwise you will exceed the capacity of your muffin pan. Not a problem if you use silicon liners that are freestanding on a baking sheet, but otherwise this could be messy and problematic.

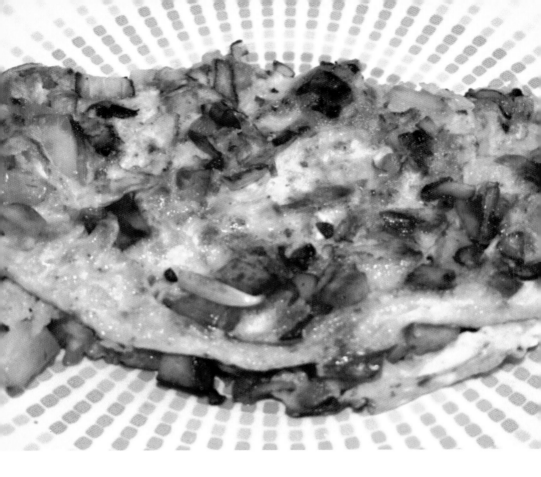

1 tablespoon butter
¼ small sweet onion
1 clove garlic, crushed
2 slices ham, finely diced
½ teaspoon salt
¼ teaspoon ground black pepper
1 teaspoon dried parsley
3 eggs, cracked and whisked together
½ cup shredded Monterrey Jack cheese

Oniony Ham Omelet

Here is one of my all time favorite omelets. There is something about the combination of onions, garlic, Monterrey Jack cheese, and eggs that just makes me happy.

Prep Time: 8 minutes

Cook Time: 15 minutes

Servings: 1-2

In medium skillet, melt butter over medium high heat. Add onion and garlic. Sauté for a few minutes until they begin to sweat. Add ham and cook until ham, garlic and onions begin to brown. Add salt, pepper and parsley. Lower heat to medium low.

Spread out ham mixture in pan. Pour in egg and swirl pan around to spread it out. Sprinkle cheese over the egg all the way to the edge. Let cook covered for about five minutes until egg sets. Using a spatula, pull egg in from the edges of the pan. When egg from the middle of the pan begins to bubble, slide your spatula under half of it and quickly flip it over the other half of the egg, pushing a little from the middle to complete the folding in half.

Cover and cook for another two minute until the egg is to desired doneness. Serve immediately.

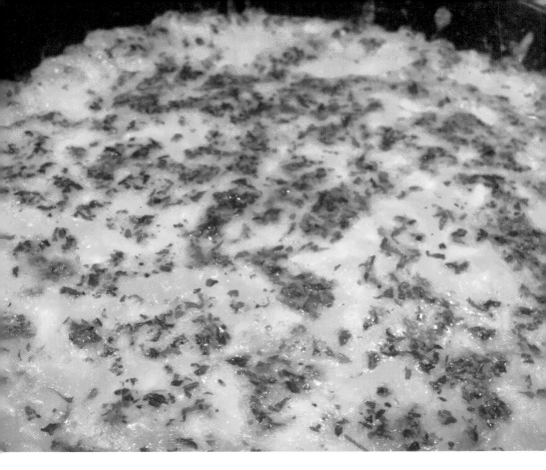

1 tablespoon extra virgin olive oil
½ pound spicy or regular breakfast sausage
½ medium yellow onion, chopped
2 garlic cloves, minced
½ large turnip, finely chopped (optional)
1 teaspoon salt (you may need more or less, depending
   on saltiness of the sausage)
½ teaspoon ground black pepper
1 tablespoon dried parsley flakes
1 tablespoon dried basil leaves
1 tablespoon dried oregano leaves
1½ cups eggs, cracked
2 tablespoons heavy whipping cream
1 cup shredded co-jack cheese

Sausage Herb Frittata

Frittatas are such an appealing dish when we have a busy day. Meats and vegetables go together so well in so many combinations, it is easy to combine them and bind with eggs. They are honorable, filling dishes that help me significantly reduce possible food waste, the thought of which makes me sad.

Prep Time: 10 minutes

Cook Time: 35 minutes

Servings: 8

Preheat oven to 300 degrees. In a 10" iron skillet*, heat the oil over medium high heat. Add onion, garlic and turnip. Sauté about four minutes until onions are translucent and garlic is browning. Add sausage, stir and cook for about five minutes until sausage is heated through.

While sausage is heating up, combine eggs into a medium bowl with salt, pepper, parsley, basil, oregano and cream. Whisk together until egg whites and yolks are well combined.

Remove skillet from heat.

Pour egg mixture over contents of skillet and stir until egg mixture and sausage/vegetable mixture are well combined. Sprinkle cheese on top of the egg, sprinkling a little more parsley, basil and oregano if you like.

Place skillet on the middle rack of the oven. Bake for 20 minutes. Move skillet to top rack and bake for ten more minutes (or it can remain on the middle rack for a more lightly browned top). Remove from oven. The center of the frittattta should be a little puffy. Let sit for about five minutes before serving—the puffiness will settle while it cools. Carefully remove full frittata from pan to serving dish, or serve directly from the iron skillet.

*This frittata can be made in an oven-proof baking dish if you don't have the noted iron skillet size. Just make sure it is no larger than 10"x10" to ensure the mixture is thick enough to prevent drying out when it is baked thoroughly. If an iron skillet is not used, additional baking time may be needed (about 5-8 minutes), since iron skillets speed up cooking time.

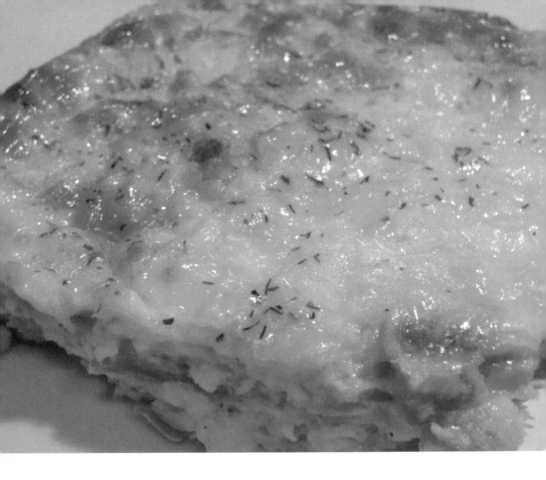

1½ cups eggs
½ cup heavy cream
1½ teaspoon dill weed
½ teaspoon salt
¼ teaspoon ground black pepper
Dash dried red chili flakes
4 ounces smoked or poached salmon, roughly
   chopped
3 slices cooked bacon, crumbled
1 cup Colby jack cheese, grated
½ cup mozzarella cheese, grated

Simple Salmon Frittata

I get very used to tossing onion and garlic into many morning egg dishes, but I also leave them out sometimes, depending on the ingredients. This time I chose to let the salmon sing without the other stronger flavors, and it did!

Prep Time: 15 minutes

Cook Time: 40 minutes (plus 10 minutes cooling)

Servings: 6

Preheat oven to 350 degrees.

Crack eggs into a medium bowl and whisk until slightly frothy. Whisk in cream, salt, pepper, chili flakes and 1 teaspoon of dill. Grease a 9x9 baking or pie dish. An iron skillet can be used as well, but you will need to reduce baking time by 5-8 minutes.

Pour in egg mixture. Sprinkle salmon and bacon evenly into the egg mixture. It should sink down into the egg. Follow the fish and bacon with the Colby Jack cheese and then mozzarella cheese. Spread the last of the dill weed and a bit more salt on top. Bake for 30-40 minutes, until edges are browning, middle egg is set and middle cheese is slightly bubbly. Remove from oven and let sit for about ten minutes. Slice and serve.

SOUPS

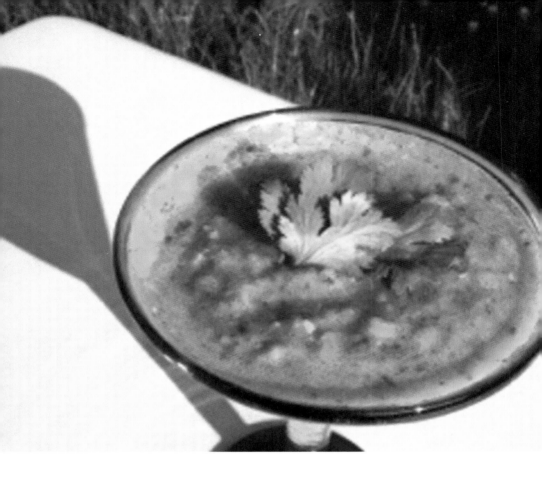

2 pounds ripe tomatoes, trimmed and
  coarsely chopped
1 small cucumber, peeled and seeded
½ red bell pepper, seeded and chopped
3 garlic cloves, crushed
½ cup parsley, loosely packed
½ sweet Vidalia onion, coarsely chopped
½ teaspoon salt
⅛ - ¼ cup sherry

Gazpacho

As summer arrives every year, I eagerly await fresh, local tomatoes. They are big, deep red and delicious. I love throwing them in a blender with other ingredients, then waiting a bit for the flavors to merge.

Prep Time: 20 minutes

Cook Time: 0 (plus 2 hours chilling)

Servings: 7 (1 cup each)

Combine all ingredients except sherry into a blender or food processor. Pulse until just combined and all pieces are of uniform size.

Add ⅛ cup sherry and pulse again to combine. If you like chunkier soup, don't pulse further. For smoother soup, continue pulsing to a smooth texture, and follow up with straining the soup through a sieve.

Depending on the sweetness of the tomatoes and onion, you may need more sherry and/or salt. If you are not sure, chill soup for about an hour and taste before deciding.

Chill at least two hours or overnight before serving. Garnish individual servings with any combination of tomato/cucumber/bell pepper/herbs you wish.

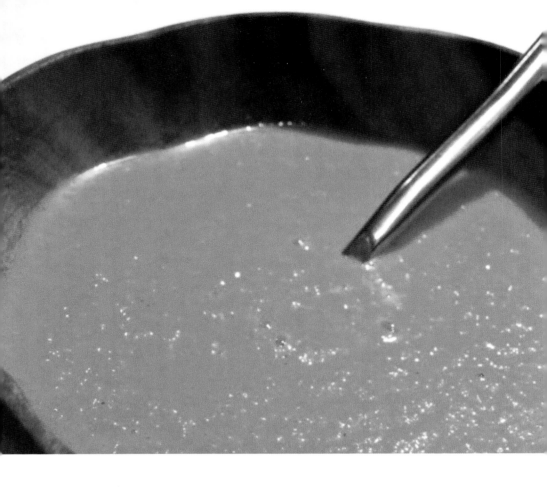

42-45 ounces diced tomatoes with juice
¼ cup red wine or beef/chicken broth
2 cloves garlic, crushed
¼ cup chopped onion
1 stalk celery, chopped
½ teaspoon salt
Dash ground black pepper
¼ teaspoon turmeric
¼ cup heavy whipping cream
Additional salt to taste

Simple Tomato Soup

One of my daughter's favorite restaurant soups is tomato. There are a number of places that offer it regularly, so she often seeks it out. At home I will whip up a batch of it when she has a hankering. I often vary it a bit, depending what is in the fridge, but this is the basic tasty recipe, including bunches of veggies and some cream for fat. She slurps it up and always gives me a big thank you smile. The greatest thing ever.

Prep Time: 10 minutes

Cook Time: 35 minutes

Servings: 9 (1 cup each)

In medium pot over medium-high heat, add all ingredients except cream. Cover and cook until bubbly, about five minutes. Stir, reduce heat to low and cover. Simmer for 30 minutes, until onions and celery are soft.

Turn off heat and let cool for about ten minutes. Add cream and stir.

Using a stick blender, puree the soup until smooth. Alternately, put soup in a blender and puree until smooth. Serve immediately, or reheat without boiling.

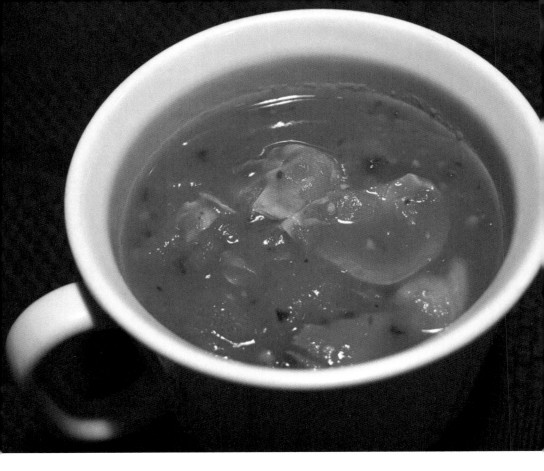

29-30 ounce can diced tomatoes with juice, or 4 cups
fresh

29-30 ounce can tomato sauce, or 4 cups fresh

1 14.5 ounce can whole medium artichoke hearts,
drained

1 cup chicken broth

½ medium onion, diced

1 tablespoon finely chopped fresh basil

2 cloves garlic

1 pinch red pepper flakes

1/16 teaspoon pure stevia powder (equivalent to one
teaspoon pure cane sugar)

1 tablespoon Worcestershire sauce

Salt and Pepper to taste

Tomato Artichoke Soup

Served along with grilled cheese or egg salad sandwiches, this soup makes for a wonderful dinner from the pantry. Fresh is always better, but sometimes there is a lack of time. I did not use cream this time to smooth out the soup's texture, but if you add ½ to ¾ cup during the last half of the cooking process the soup can only get better.

Prep Time: 10 minutes

Cook Time: 1 hour, 10 minutes

Servings: 6 (2 cups each)

Break up artichoke hearts into bite-sized pieces and separate by gently pushing on them with a soup spoon.

Combine all ingredients except salt into a medium pot over medium high heat. Bring soup to a boil. Lower temperature and cover, simmering for about an hour. Adjust flavor with salt as desired.

Serve immediately or chill and reheat on low before serving.

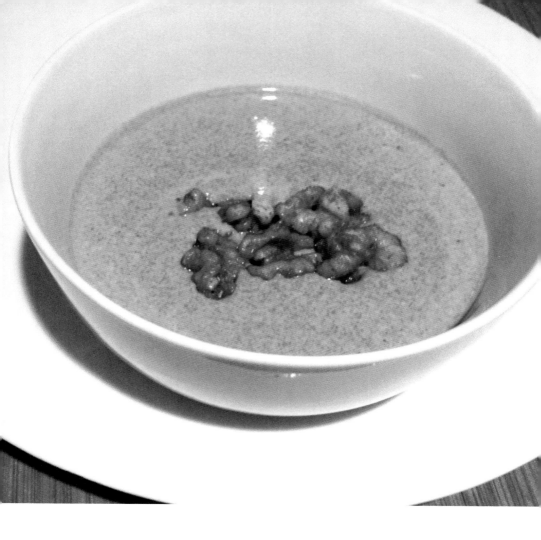

3 tablespoons butter or oil
4 cloves garlic, crushed
¼ sweet onion, finely chopped
6 cups fresh baby spinach
1 cup chicken stock
3 ounces cream cheese
3 ounces beer (I recommend an IPA), or use
   extra broth as a substitute
1 cup heavy cream
½ cup Parmesan cheese
Nuts as garnish (I recommend roasted or
   savory spiced nuts)

Spinach Soup

I like green veggies. Ever since I was a kid I especially liked spinach when the other kids thought 'yech'! My mom once told me a story about, me, my brother and spinach. We went to daycare when we were little, and one day when we came home we would not eat our spinach. Apparently we were told by other kids we were not supposed to like it, so we did not eat it. Talk about peer pressure! We eventually succumbed and joyfully continued to eat it, but we did have that blip.

Since spinach is still a favored vegetable, I of course had to come up with a great soup that included it! Savory and filling, it is a wonderful thing. The soup freezes and reheats well, so is also a great lunch addition.

Prep Time: 10 minutes

Cook Time: 30 minutes

Servings: 8 (1 cup each)

In large sauce pot, melt butter over medium heat. Add garlic and onion, cooking until they begin to brown.

Add spinach and toss until it wilts and begins to darken, about five minutes.

Add beer and simmer until soup is hot.

Add cream cheese, heavy cream, and Parmesan cheese, and stir. Continue cooking until the cheese is melted.

Using a hand blender, puree until spinach is macerated and soup is smooth. Simmer on low for about five minutes.

Sprinkle individual servings with nuts and serve immediately.

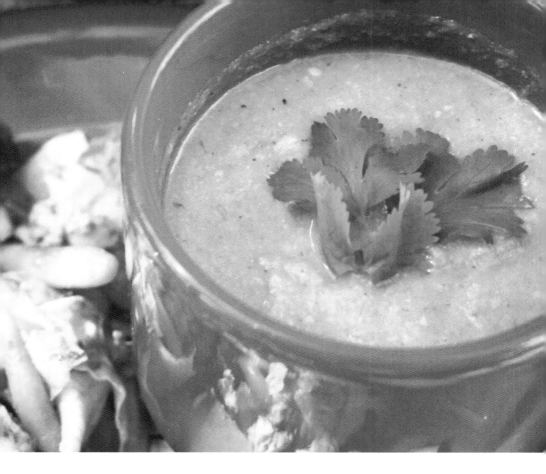

1 cup broccoli, chopped
2 cups cauliflower, chopped
3 large carrots, chopped
½ onion, chopped
1 small turnip, peeled and chopped
1 apple, chopped
1 medium tomato, chopped
2 cloves garlic, chopped
5 cups chicken broth
2 teaspoons dried thyme leaves
1 teaspoon ground sage
2 teaspoons dried parsley leaves
2 teaspoons salt
1 dash cayenne pepper
2 tablespoons olive oil

Prep Time: 20 minutes

Cook Time: 1 hour

Servings: 10 (1 cup each)

Dancing Vegetable Soup

I called this dish dancing vegetable soup because it made me dance when I made it. I was in a rush and pureed the soup while it was still over the heat. I have done this before, and did not think twice about doing it this time, but I failed to turn the heat down. Having the heat on is fine, but having it too high is downright dangerous. Oops!

When the soup was half pureed, some bubbles rose from the bottom (trying to get away from all that heat underneath it). The evil bubbles splashed steaming hot soup onto my left thumb where I was holding the pot and also the bottom of the wrist of my right hand that was holding the stick blender. I popped back away from the stove and did a twisty spin while flailing my arms about as I headed to the sink. The soup was thick and clung to my skin. It really hurt.

As I ran cold water on my hand and wrist, I did a kind of jogging side step, then lunged for the freezer to get a cold pack. As the cold pack cooled off my hot skin my daughter woke up from her nap, crying from a bad dream, so on the way to the bedroom to soothe her I was balancing the pack between my left hand and the bottom of my right wrist. It was slippery.

After I got my girl calmed down, she asked me what the cold pack was for. I told her I burned myself and showed here where it happened. She kissed my burn spots and they felt a lot better.

As you can see from the ingredient list, this soup is high in fiber and low fat (by accident). It tastes great hot or cold. I usually only eat about a cup along with a sandwich or salad, because it is pretty filling.

Heat oil at medium high in a large pot. Add onion and garlic, cooking them until they sweat and sear a bit. Add remaining vegetables and stir to spread onions and garlic throughout. Add broth, salt and spices.

Cover and simmer until vegetables are cooked soft, about 45 minutes, or in a pressure cooker for ten minutes with natural release.

Remove from heat. Puree soup with an immersion blender until smooth.

Return to heat and simmer for 10 more minutes. Serve hot or cold.

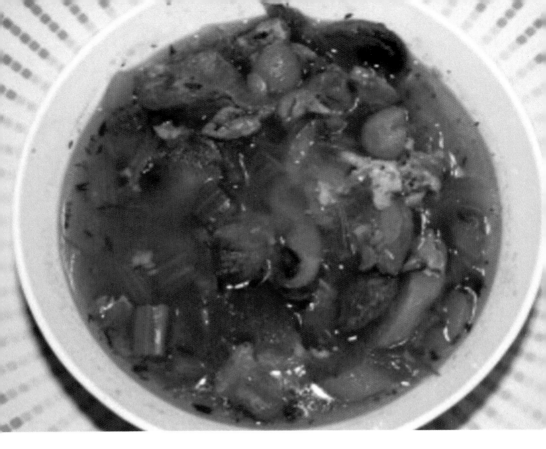

½ pound thick sliced mushrooms

3 tablespoons dried thyme

1 teaspoon salt

2 tablespoons extra virgin olive oil

3 limes, juiced with meat included

2 pounds cooked chicken, chopped or shredded

2 cups petite carrots, chopped into coins

3 stalks celery, chopped

1 medium onion, chopped

4 cloves garlic, crushed

4 small or roma tomatoes, roughly chopped

3 cups water

12 ounces beer* (pick a strongly flavored one—pale ale or IPA goes well with the lime)

Salt to taste

Prep Time: 30 minutes

Cook Time: 2-10 hours, depending on cooking method

Servings: 8-10 (2 cups each)

*To fully avoid alcohol in the recipe, you can substitute chicken broth and ¼ cup apple cider vinegar for the beer. It will result in a similar tang that works with the lime juice.

Thyme and Lime Chicken Soup

You are walking along, enjoying the crisp fall breeze, when you suddenly have an urge for a bowl of hot chicken soup. You run by the store and into the soup aisle, only to discover that all their offerings include noodles, rice, tons of salt, preservatives, and fillers. Where, oh where, is the veggie- and chicken-filled bowl of goodness you were craving? And what about that extra twist you want to be surprised with as the first spoonful slides down your throat? Well, here are all the things you're looking for!

The surprise in this soup is how wonderfully the beer mixes with the lime juice and thyme to give the soup a nip not usually found in chicken soup. Don't worry. After exposure to heat the alcohol cooks away, but the more subtle flavors of the beer stay in the soup.

In a medium bowl combine the juice and pulp from one lime, olive oil, thyme and salt. Add the mushrooms and toss until coated. In a pan over medium high heat cook the mushrooms until they sweat and begin until brown. Remove from heat and set aside to cool.

CROCKPOT METHOD: In crock pot add water and remaining lime juice with pulp, then turn pot to high. Add chicken, carrots, celery, onion, garlic and tomatoes. Stir and let soup heat up, about an hour.

When the soup is hot add chicken, mushrooms (along with any of their juices) and the beer to the pot. Continue to cook on high for three more hours. Turn temperature to low and cook for 3–4 more hours.

All the ingredients can be added to the crock pot at the same time and cooked on low for 8–10 hours, but the resulting soup is tangier if the vegetables are allowed to heat up in the water/lime liquid before adding the beer. Either method bears good results.

STOVETOP METHOD: If using the stovetop, bring the soup to a boil before adding the mushrooms and beer, then simmer on low for 4 hours. Season with salt to taste before serving.

PRESSURE COOKER METHOD: If using a pressure cooker to prepare the soup, cook all of the ingredients at the same time for 30 minutes at pressure with natural release.

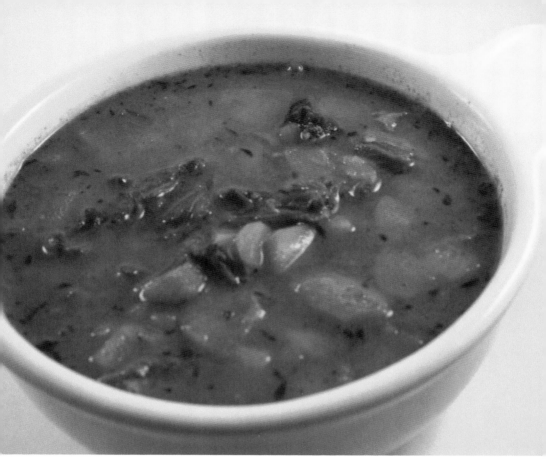

1 pound oxtail, cut into 2-inch thick
  slices
3 tablespoons oil
¾ cup red wine (can be excluded if
  alcohol is a concern)
3 garlic cloves, cut in half
8 cups water
1 teaspoon salt
1 teaspoon ground ginger
2 large carrots, diced
1 medium turnip, diced
1 large or 2 small onions, diced
3 stalks celery, diced
2 small potatoes, diced (can be
  excluded or increase turnip quantity)
2 teaspoons chopped thyme
1 teaspoon chopped parsley
Salt and Pepper to taste

Oxtail Soup

My dad learned how to make oxtail soup in Germany where, as in most areas of the world, every bit and piece of slaughtered animals is used. It has a rich sauce and the vegetables melt in your mouth. He would leave the meat on the bones and we would each get one in our bowl. As a kid it was fun trying to get all the meat out of the little crevasses.

The dog was always hanging around while we ate it, trying to wait patiently for the bones.

Oxen have meaty tails, and the meat is pretty tender. Of course, most meat is tender after being cooked for three hours. The oxtail is traditionally considered one of the more lowly cuts of meat. I mean, you don't typically find oxtails on the menu of fine dining establishments, but in many places of the world soup made with them is very popular. The marrow adds extra depth of flavor to the broth. The meat and simple vegetables in the soup are relied on to warm bellies on cold winter nights.

Prep Time: Day 1, 20 minutes. Day 2, 30 minutes

Cook Time: Day 1, 3 ½ hours. Day 2, 1-3 hours depending on cooking method

Servings: 9 (2 cups each)

The day before making the soup, the oxtail pieces need to be cooked. In a deep pan on the stovetop (I used a dutch oven) heat the oil, add the oxtail pieces, and sear on all sides. Add the salt, garlic, water and wine, and scrape the brown bits off the bottom of the pot. Bring it to a boil then lower heat, cover and let simmer for about three hours.

A pressure cooker can be used with one hour pressure time and natural release, but make sure the searing is done thoroughly prior.

When cooking is complete, the meat should be falling off the bones. Let cool until the meat can be handled and remove the tails from the broth. If you are going to exclude the bones from the final soup this is the time to remove as much meat as possible from the bones. Discard the bones or give them to the dogs.

Store the bones/meat and broth separately in the refrigerator overnight.

The next day, skim off/remove as much fat and garlic as you can from the broth and discard. The broth will mostly be in a gelatinous form, but will liquefy when heated. The end result of this soup is very brothy, so if too much fat is left in the final soup it can be greasy.

Return broth and bones/meat to the stovetop pot (or a crock pot), then add all the vegetables, meat and herbs. If the liquid is not covering all the vegetables you may need to add a cup or so of water or beef broth, but wait until it is warm because it might not be necessary.

Simmer on low for about three hours until the vegetables are tender (or six hours in a crock pot). If using a pressure cooker, use pressure for one hour and natural release.

Add salt and pepper to taste. Serve hot.

SALADS

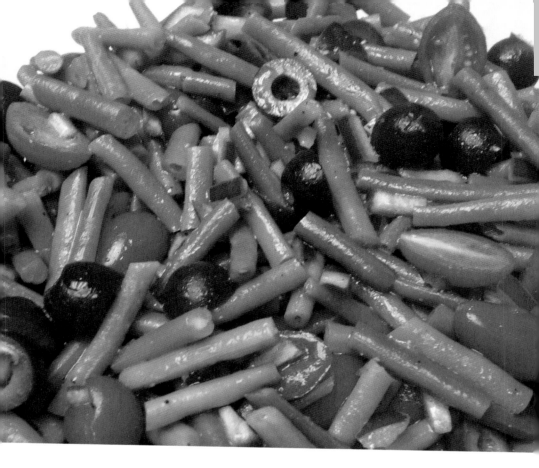

2 pounds fresh green beans
2 cups grape or small cherry tomatoes
¼ large red onion
2 cups large black olives, drained
2 cups vinaigrette dressing (see Herby
  Dressing recipe in the Dressing
  section)
Salt and Pepper to taste
2 teaspoons dried red pepper flakes
  (optional)

Prep Time: 30 minutes

**Cook Time: 0 (4 hours
  chilling)**

**Servings: 26 (½ cup
  each)**

Cold Green Bean Salad

As I have mentioned many times before, we make sure there are prepared foods stocked in our refrigerator, since there are few convenience foods that fit our sugar free, grain free eating habits. We prepare boiled eggs, bite-sized raw vegetables, cured meats and salads of all kinds. Making salads out of staples is also an easy way to keep the fridge full.

On day four after making this salad, the acids in the dressing may have made the green beans a little less bright, but the beans also soaked up all the flavors, including the tang of the red onion, and a serving of it tastes heavenly.

I encourage you to experiment with other salad fixings too! I've made similar salads using slender asparagus instead of green beans, Greek olives instead of black, mushrooms along with tomatoes, and even thrown in some chopped up ham or salami. Noticing a variation on a theme? The thing I have learned making cold salads over the years is that two cups of dressing seems to be just right to coat 9-10 cups of salad, which is the case here.

Have fun in your kitchen and enjoy the bright, healthy produce of spring!

Make your vinaigrette dressing of choice, if not already made or using store bought. Set aside.

Remove ends from green beans and slice them into bite sized pieces, about one inch. In a medium pot with steamer, insert bring one inch of salty water to a boil. Add beans to steamer and lightly steam about five minutes, with the intention to soften them but retain their bright green color. Remove beans from pot, set them aside to cool and prepare remaining ingredients.

Slice tomatoes in half lengthwise and place in bowl. Finely chop red onion and place in bowl. Slice black olives in half horizontally and place in bowl. Add green beans. If including red pepper flakes add them now.

Pour dressing over salad ingredients. Gently toss salad until well coated. Cover bowl and chill for at least four hours, or overnight.

Remove from refrigerator and toss salad again, then taste and add salt and pepper to enhance dressing flavor (need will vary depending on dressing used). Toss one more time to incorporate salt and pepper, then serve.

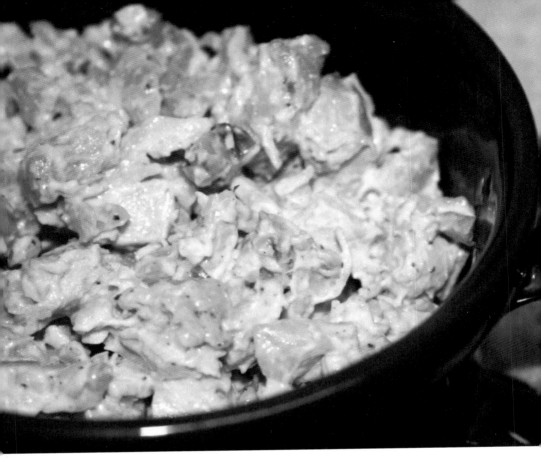

6 cups dark or white uncooked chicken, boneless and
  skinless*
2 tablespoons olive oil
1–2 tablespoons broth retained from cooking the
  chicken*
1 cup mayonnaise (in Sauces)
1 teaspoon cumin powder
1 cup raw walnuts, chopped
Salt to taste

*If you are using previously cooked chicken, either use the juices from
that chicken or water.

Walnut Chicken Salad

If you have ever been to Washington DC, you probably noticed in almost every government and office building there is a little cafe on the bottom floor. These little cafes can be addictive. They usually have delicious breakfast and lunch buffets that are sold by the pound, and are extremely convenient.

You get your little to-go container and pick bits and pieces from the display of food. A little cucumber salad, a bit of roast chicken, a spoonful of sautéed green beans, a pile of fruit, and avocado chunks.

I scooped up some chicken salad at one of the cafes. I expected it to be pleasant, like most food bar choices tend to be, but boy was I surprised. The light brown bits mixed with the chicken weren't pieces of fruit like I expected, but walnuts!

The slightly sweet taste I expected ended up being a nutty, savory flavor that blended wonderfully with the dressing and chicken. I don't know what was actually in that salad, but I ate the rest of it slowly, savoring each bite and trying to figure out what else was in there. I think I've pieced together a pretty good replica of my lunchtime discovery, which is a good thing, because I don't live in DC anymore...

Prep Time: 10 minutes

Cook Time: 10 minutes (plus chilling time)

Servings: 6 (1 cup each)

Chop chicken into bite sized pieces. Heat oil over medium high heat in a large skillet. Add chicken and toss until cooked through and browning, about ten minutes. Remove from heat and set aside to cool. Prepare the rest of the salad.

In a medium mixing bowl combine mayonnaise, cumin and walnuts. Add some of the broth to thin out the mixture to the consistency of thick salad dressing. Add chicken and toss with dressing. Chill at least two hours or overnight before serving.

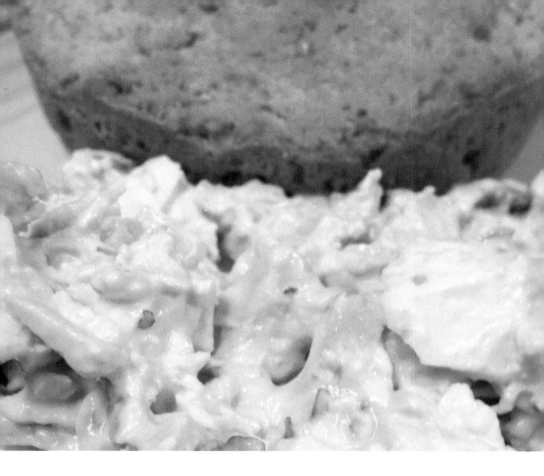

3 large chicken breasts, bone in and skin on (or
  6 cups precooked chicken)
3 boiled eggs, chopped (ten minutes boiled, or 3
  minutes pressure cooker, quick release)
3 medium dill pickles, chopped
½ medium yellow onion, chopped
¼ cup yellow mustard
1 cup sour cream
1 tablespoon salt, plus extra for chicken
1 tablespoon dried parsley leaves
2 teaspoons dried oregano leaves
2 teaspoons garlic powder, plus extra for
  chicken
1 teaspoon ground black pepper

Mustard Chicken Salad

This chicken salad is nice and savory with the onion and mustard, and keeps well in the fridge for a big meal or a quick snack. It can be served with keto friendly bread or lettuce leaves when we are seeking out a full meal.

Prep Time: 15 minutes

Cook Time: 30 minutes (plus chilling time)

Servings: 8 (1 cup each)

Preheat oven to 350 degrees. Line shallow baking dish with aluminum foil.

Liberally season both sides of breasts with salt and garlic powder. Bake skin side up for 30 minutes on the top shelf of the oven. If you are using boneless skinless breasts cooking time may need to be reduced by five to ten minutes. Remove from oven and let cool. Separate bones and skin from breasts. Cut meat into bite-sized cubes. You should have 4-6 cups of chicken.

In a large bowl, whisk together the sour cream, mustard, salt, parsley, oregano, garlic powder and black pepper. Add the onion, eggs, pickle and chicken.

Fold in the dressing with the other ingredients until everything is evenly coated.

Chill for at least 30 minutes to ensure the chicken is cold. Serve with some keto friendly bread, lettuce for wrapping, or fresh vegetables.

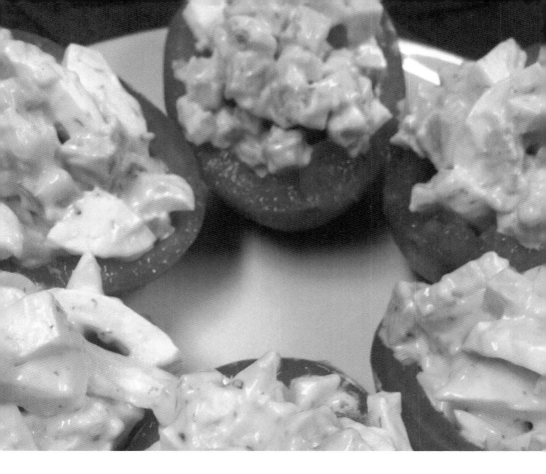

4 boiled eggs, roughly chopped (ten minutes boiled,
   or 3 minutes pressure cooker, quick release)
½ cup mayonnaise (in Sauces)
1 tablespoon yellow mustard
1 teaspoon dill leaves
½ teaspoon garlic powder
¼ teaspoon onion powder
Salt and pepper to taste
1 cup diced ham
6 roma tomatoes, halved lengthwise and seeds
   removed
Chopped chives for garnish (optional)

Ham and Egg Salad Tomatoes

I often seek out quick, oven-free meals when feasible, especially during the summer. Spying the ever-present boiled eggs, ham and tomatoes in the fridge, I came up with a fun idea. Stuffed tomatoes! The same staple foods we often eat, but in a different little package! I have done something similar with tuna and cherry tomatoes, for a dainty tea party dish, but never used egg salad or larger roma tomatoes before. These would go great as make ahead for a luncheon or pot luck.

Prep Time: 20 minutes

Cook Time: 0

Servings: 12

In a medium bowl, combine mayonnaise, mustard, garlic powder, onion powder, dill leaves, and a dash of salt and pepper. Whisk together until well combined.

Add eggs and ham. Stir until ham and egg are coated.

Fill each tomato half with salad, mounding it on top and gently pressing it into the hollow of the tomato. Place on platter, sprinkle with chives, and serve immediately, or cover and refrigerate until served.

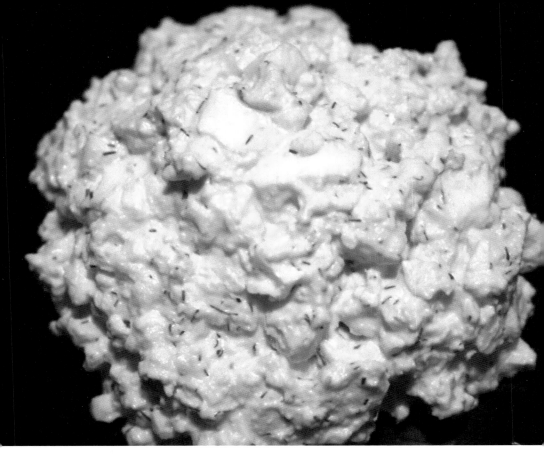

12 eggs, hard boiled and peeled (ten minutes
   boiled, or 3 minutes pressure cooker, quick
   release)
½ cup mayonnaise (see Sauce section for
   recipe)
1 tablespoon yellow mustard
1 tablespoon dried dill weed
½ teaspoon salt
1 teaspoon garlic powder
½ teaspoon onion powder

Dilly Egg Salad

I know this is a very simple recipe that almost everyone can do without direction, but it is still nice to write it down, put it together, and enjoy the results. It is great to know the basics so you can then get all creative and add your own personal twists.

Prep Time: 15 minutes

Cook Time: 0 (plus chilling)

Servings: 6

Combine all ingredients except eggs and whisk together. Add eggs to dressing and dice by using two sharp knives in a crisscross motion. Make them chunky or finely mashed as you like. Stir until all egg bits are coated with dressing.

Cover and refrigerate at least an hour before serving.

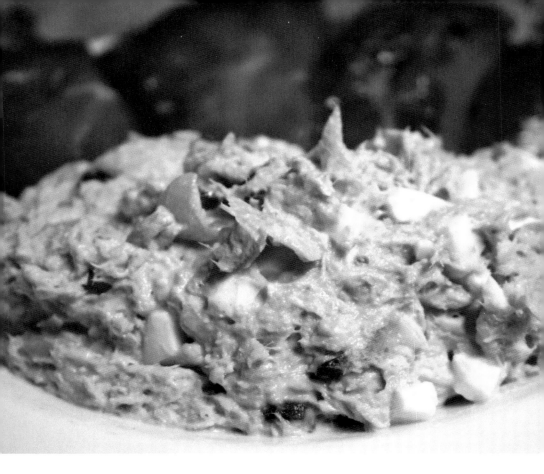

1 pound tuna in water (about four small cans)
4 boiled eggs (ten minutes boiled, or 3 minutes
   pressure cooker, quick release)
1 teaspoon olive oil
½ small sweet onion, finely chopped
4 garlic cloves, finely chopped
½ cup mayonnaise (in Sauces)
2 tablespoons horseradish mustard (or 1½
   tablespoons mustard, 2 teaspoons raw
   horseradish)
Salt and Pepper to taste

Tuna Salad Sauté

The word sauté may sound like a hot dish, but after the sautéed portion of this salad cools off and is chilled, you won't think of sautéing the same again. The sweetness of the onion and garlic work really well with the tuna and egg.

Prep Time: 20 minutes

Cook Time: 0 (plus at least an hour for chilling)

Servings: 8

Heat oil in small pan over medium heat. Add onion and garlic. Sauté until browned and beginning to caramelize. Set aside to cool while the rest of the salad is prepared.

Drain water from tuna into small bowl. Place tuna in a mixing bowl and serve drained tuna liquid to eager cats.

Roughly chop eggs and add them to the tuna.

Add mayonnaise, mustard, salt and pepper to tuna. Stir ingredients until mixed. Add onion and garlic, and stir some more until all the large pieces are pretty evenly distributed.

Chill for at least an hour before serving.

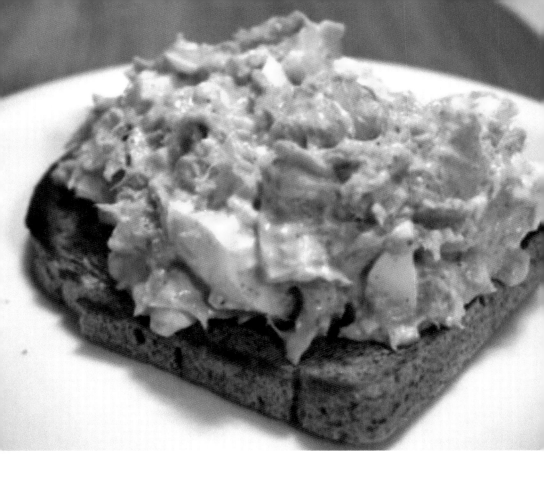

1 large ripe avocado
8–10 hard boiled eggs (ten minutes boiled, or
 3 minutes pressure cooker, quick release)
1 5-ounce can tuna packed in water, drained
½ cup Greek yogurt or sour cream*
2 tablespoons lime juice
1 teaspoon stone ground mustard
½ teaspoon salt
½ teaspoon ground cumin
¼ teaspoon chili powder
Sprinkle of ground black pepper

Don't Have To Choose Salad

Do I want egg salad, tuna salad, or guacamole? To take full advantage of my indecisiveness I decided to combine them all. I wanted the flavor of all three to be present and also work together. Tuna is a great way to add protein to a dish, even if there are already protein and healthy fats eking out of the avocado and egg.

Prep Time: 15 minutes

Cook Time: 0 (plus chilling)

Servings: 6

In a large bowl, whisk together yogurt, juice, mustard, salt, cumin, chili powder and pepper. Roughly chop eggs and avocado into pieces about the same size. Gently fold the tuna, avocado and eggs with the dressing, trying not to crush the pieces.
Chill for about an hour before serving.

*For a dairy free dish, substitute unsweetened coconut cream from a chilled can of whole fat coconut milk - when a can of coconut milk is chilled the solids rise, so it can be scooped out while the coconut water stays at the bottom of the can.

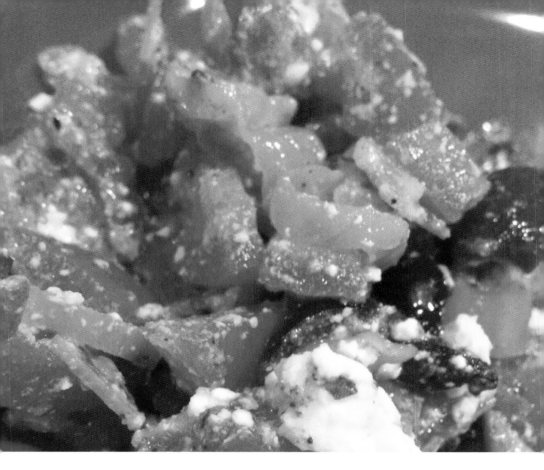

1 cup mixed green, black and kalamata olives, pitted

1 cup pepperoncini peppers, chopped

½ cup crumbled feta cheese

½ cup marinated artichoke hearts, diced

3 plum tomatoes, diced and seeds removed

¼ yellow or white onion, finely diced

4 ounces thin sliced salami or pepperoni, diced

⅓ cup vinaigrette or Herby Dressing (see Dressing Section for recipe)

Antipasto Salad

In spite of the name, antipasto does not mean it does not like pasta, but it HAS no pasta, and it comes BEFORE pasta. Just the way we like it.

Prep Time: 20 minutes

Cook Time: 0 (plus 15 minutes resting time)

Servings: 5

Roughly chop olives so they are of similar size. Place olives in medium bowl.

Add peppers, cheese, artichoke hearts, tomatoes, onion and salami. Lightly toss.

Add dressing and stir until well coated. Let sit for about 15 minutes then toss again and serve. The salad can also be made a day in advance and chilled until time to serve.

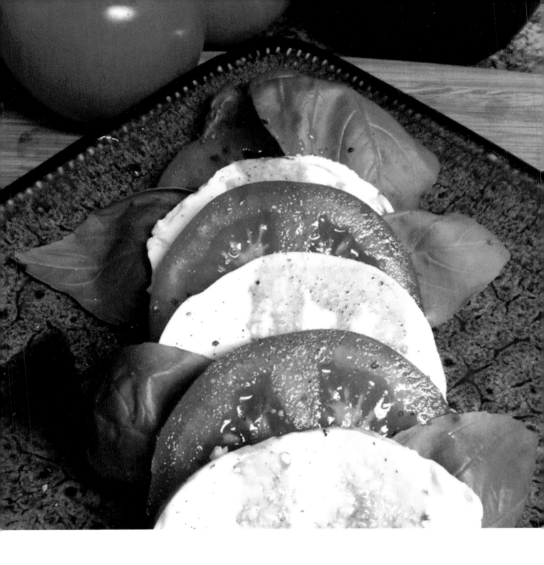

1 large red tomato
1 ball fresh mozzarella
1 large stem fresh basil
Extra virgin olive oil
Aged basalmic vinegar
Salt and Pepper to taste

Caprese Salad

When I smell basil I think of my trip to Italy, the Tuscany region. The quiet evenings, fresh steaks and veal from the local shop, and another funny and memorable element: frogs croaking in the pond below our bedroom window all night.

Believe it or not, it was like an elixir, lulling us to sleep. On to the salad.

I almost called it insalata caprese, but decided not to because of the—dum dum dum—basalmic vinegar. I loved salad when made with fresh ingredients and high quality olive oil, but don't recall ever seeing the basalmic vinegar offered in Italy, only in the US. My research was consistent. Insalata caprese is typically seasoned with salt, pepper and olive oil.

Prep Time: 10 minutes

Cook Time: 0

Servings: 4

Slice tomato and mozzarella into slices of equal thickness.
Sprinkle slices with salt and pepper.
Layer slices with leaves of basil.
Sprinkle salad with olive oil and basalmic vinegar.
Serve immediately.

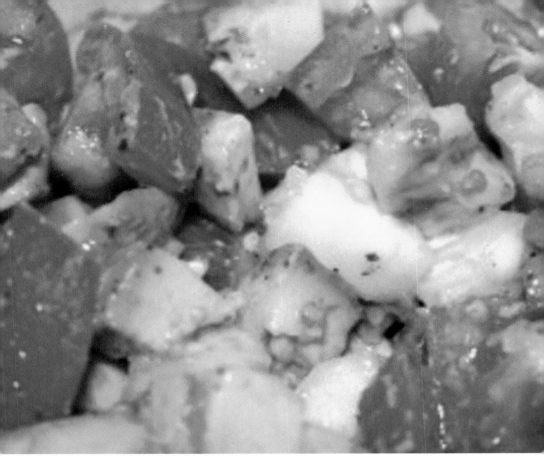

4 tablespoons extra virgin olive oil
2 tablespoons apple cider vinegar
1 small bunch basil leaves (10-12), finely chopped
1 teaspoon salt
1 teaspoon ground black pepper
½ lime, juiced with pulp
2 ripe avocados, peeled and coarsely chopped
3 roma tomatoes, cut into about 20 pieces each
½ large cucumber, seeds removed, peeled and
  coarsely chopped

End Of Summer Salad

Here is a wonderful, simple, soft salad that fully appreciates some of the local Texas summer fruits and vegetables.

When temperatures gently creep lower in Autumn I tend to linger over the fresh, seasonal summer produce at the markets. I know some of it, although sadder looking, will be around pretty much year round by importing to grocery stores from all over the world. Some will have faded colors or less flavor. Others will just get more expensive.

I look forward to the local squash and root vegetables that are still around in September, but I always cherish the last of the bright local tomatoes, abundant cucumber, and basil that have become a summer habit over the years.

Prep Time: 15 minutes

Cook Time: 0 (plus chilling)

Servings: 6

In a small bowl combine the first six ingredients. Set aside.

In a large bowl combine the avocado, tomato and cucumber. Add dressing and stir gently, trying not to smash tomatoes or avocado too much.

Chill covered for about an hour before serving.

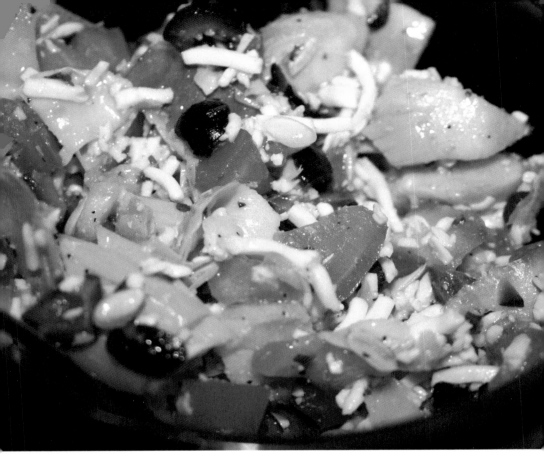

3 tablespoons apple cider vinegar
1 teaspoon salt*
½ teaspoon ground black pepper
1 tablespoon dried parsley leaves
1 teaspoon garlic powder
½ teaspoon onion powder
Dash of dried red pepper flakes
4 tablespoons extra virgin olive oil
2 medium tomatoes, rough chopped
½ large cucumber (or zucchini), rough chopped
1 cup artichoke hearts, rough chopped
½ cup chopped black olives
1 cup shredded Monterrey Jack, feta or Parmesan
  cheese

Another End Of Summer Salad

I have to say right now that I absolutely adore my daughter. Now I must also say that I really enjoyed making this salad all by myself—not having to lean over a footstool, without a helper who is learning to use a knife, or a munchkin putting a little too much parsley in the bowl, or an imp who insists on measuring and pouring the olive oil from the huge bottle on her own and spilling about half a cup on the counter.

While she watched the last bit of *Willy Wonka and the Chocolate Factory* (the 1971 version, thank you very much), I snuck into the kitchen and whipped up this salad. I liked doing it by myself as much as I will enjoy the next time she helps me break a dozen eggs for a frittata—it's just a different way of cooking.

Prep Time: 20 minutes

Cook Time: 0

Servings: 6

Add first seven ingredients in small bowl. While whisking the vinegar mixture, gradually add olive oil until well combined.

In a medium bowl, add tomatoes, cucumber/zucchini, artichoke hearts, olives, and cheese. Drizzle dressing over vegetables and gently stir until it is evenly distributed.

Chill for at least 20 minutes. Toss again before serving.

*If you use feta or Parmesan cheese you may need less than 1 teaspoon of salt, since they tend to be stronger, salty cheeses.

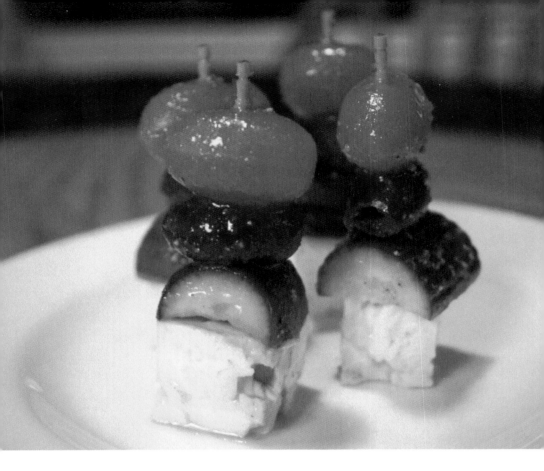

24 toothpicks
1 8-ounce block feta cheese, cut into 24 cubes
24 grape tomatoes
24 kalamata olives, pitted
1 English cucumber or 3 mini cucumbers
½ medium red onion, large rough chopped (optional)
¼ cup olive oil
⅛ cup red wine or balsamic vinegar
1 teaspoon lemon juice
½ teaspoon salt
¼ teaspoon pepper
1 teaspoon dried oregano

Greek Salad On A Stick

Greek salads are things I can just eat and eat, especially with some hot grilled beef or chicken kebabs on top.

I have made these wonderful little appetizers a number of times and love the juiciness with the dressing added. The whole stick of salad can fit in one bite. Whoa! Heaven!

Sometimes I include onion, but usually not because some of my nearest and dearest have a hard time with raw onion. But it definitely adds a layer of flavor if you choose to do so.

Prep Time: 30 minutes

Cook Time: 0 (plus 1 hour chilling)

Servings: 24

Whisk together the last six ingredients. Set aside.

Slice cucumbers into thick slices, about ½ inch in length, then again in half or quarters, depending on cucumber size. As you can see in the picture, the radius of the cucumber pieces should be about as thick as the tomatoes.

I have found that all four elements' successfullty fitting on the toothpicks is directly related to the size of the four elements (especially the squishiness of the olives, but that can only go so far), so do a test 'pick before cutting up all the cucumber.

Start with putting on toothpicks the tomato, followed by an olive and cucumber, ending with the feta. Place all the filled toothpicks in a deep plate or bowl that will just hold the completed 'picks. If including onion sprinkle pieces over the top of the toothpicks, so the pieces fall randomly among the toothpicks.

Drizzle dressing over the 'picks. Refrigerate for at least an hour. Before serving move the 'picks to a serving dish, standing on the base of the feta square and again drizzle the dressing over the 'picks. The onion can be served on the side.

If you use fancy decorated 'picks, the tops of which won't look good when slimed with dressing, you may need to spoon the dressing over them to avoid the fancy parts.

VEGETABLES

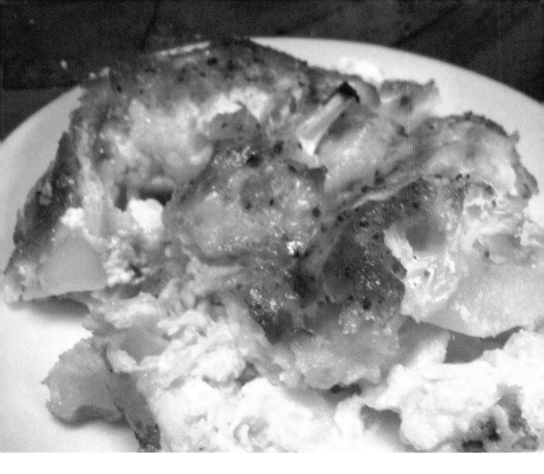

1 head cauliflower
2 eggs
1 cup heavy whipping cream
1 tablespoon salt, plus more for top
1 teaspoon ground black pepper, plus more for top
1 teaspoon onion powder, plus more for top
1 teaspoon garlic powder, plus more for top
2 cups grated sharp cheddar cheese
1½ cups grated parmigiana reggiano cheese

Cauliflower and Cheese

This time was different. This time it worked just right. There were chewiness, cheesiness, and creaminess that worked like a comfort food. That reminded me of the mac n cheese of my youth.

Sometimes ham or hot dogs were chopped up with it and made it even more salty. The taste of this meal also reminded me of meatless Fridays that were part of the religious aspects of my upbringing. I never actually missed the meat as I dug into the creamy cheesiness.

After a few mouthfuls, this time, my daughter asked if I would make this every night because it was "soooooo good!"

I don't know if I can accomplish that, but it certainly is not hard to do if there is a kitchen nearby and barely took more time than fixing mac n cheese from a box! It would be so cool if she craved cauliflower instead of pasta in 20 years…

Prep Time: 20 minutes

Cook Time: 45 minutes (plus 10 minutes' resting)

Servings: 10

Preheat oven to 350 degrees.

Remove leaves and stem from cauliflower. Cut cauliflower head into bite-sized pieces, keeping the florets as intact as possible to avoid crumbling.

In a medium bowl whisk the eggs and cream, then add the salt, pepper, onion powder and garlic powder. Add ½ cup of the cheddar cheese and stir in with the cream mixture.

Arrange the cauliflower evenly in a 9"x13" baking dish. Sprinkle some salt on the cauliflower. Pour the creamy cheese mixture over cauliflower. Spread the cheddar and parmigiana reggiano cheese to cover the top entirely.

Sprinkle a bit more salt, pepper, onion powder and garlic powder on top. Place uncovered in preheated oven for 40-45 minutes, until top is browned and bubbly. Remove from oven and let rest for ten minutes before serving.

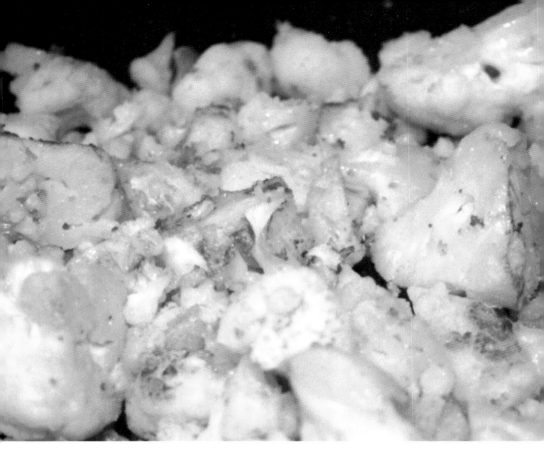

1 head cauliflower
3 tablespoons butter
2 garlic cloves, crushed
¼ teaspoon nutmeg
Salt and pepper to taste

Cauliflower Sauté

Here is another quick way to prepare cauliflower, in case you did not get enough already in this book. We eat a lot of the stuff in our home, and I doubt there's an end in sight. I swear this time it is different, and enjoy it along a spicy or busy main dish.

Nutmeg may sound like an odd spice to use outside of a dessert, but it works amazingly well with cauliflower (and cabbage, for that matter), and helps keep preparation simple and flavorful. It is pretty common in Middle Eastern and European dishes to use nutmeg in savory vegetable and meat dishes. After you use it with cauliflower you will understand why.

I like making cauliflower on the stovetop whenever the oven is busy cooking the rest of the meal. It is easy to let it basically prepare itself while I am getting other parts of the meal done, then leaving it covered off the heat keeps it warm and ready to serve.

Prep Time: 10 minutes

Cook Time: 20 minutes

Servings: 8

Cut cauliflower into bite-size florets.

In a large skillet, melt butter over medium heat. Add garlic and cook for a few minutes until it softens. Turn up heat to high and add cauliflower. Toss so the butter and garlic coat the florets.

Cook until the cauliflower begins to brown, about five minutes. Add nutmeg, salt and pepper and continue to toss every minute or so, allowing more browning.

When about half the floret surfaces are browned, turn heat to low and cover, cooking the cauliflower until preferred softness, about five to ten more minutes.

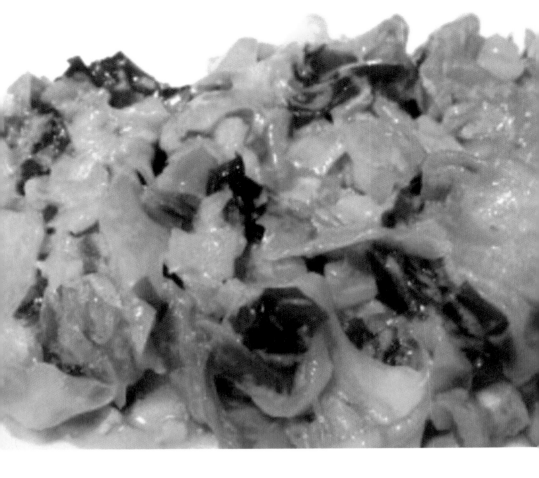

2 tablespoons butter or bacon fat
½ medium cabbage head, roughly chopped
2 - 3 cups collard greens, stems removed and
  chopped
½ cup mayonnaise (in Sauces) or
  ¼ cup heavy whipping cream
½ teaspoon red or ancho chili powder
Salt and Pepper to taste

Creamy Cabbage Collard Mix

The savory combination in this mix is a wonderful complement to a spicy meat dish and adds the requisite fiber to the meal. It is very rich and tastes almost decadent, but is still good for you!

Prep Time: 10 minutes

Cook Time: 25 minutes

Servings: 7

Heat a large frying pan to medium-high heat. Add butter and mayonnaise or cream, and chili powder. Heat until mayonnaise is melted or cream is bubbly.

Add cabbage and greens. Sprinkle generously with salt and pepper. Stir until vegetables are coated. Lower heat to medium and let cook for about ten minutes, stirring every few minutes until cabbage and greens are wilted, but still slightly crispy.

Remove from heat and cover until time to serve.

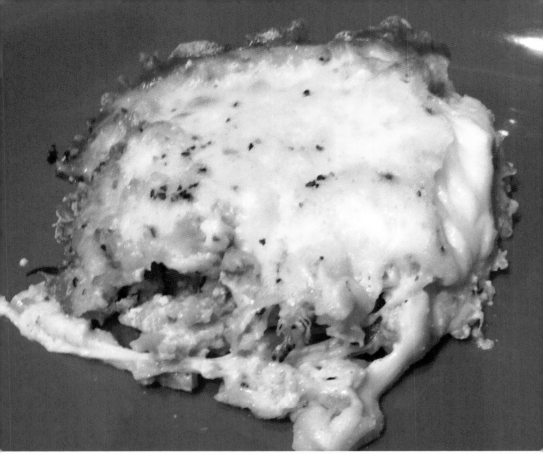

1 small head cauliflower
1 stalk broccoli
½ small onion
2 eggs
1 cup heavy whipping cream
1 teaspoon salt
1 teaspoon ground black pepper
2 teaspoons granulated garlic
½ teaspoon ground thyme
2 tablespoons lemon juice
3 cups shredded mozzarella cheese

Cheesy White And Green Bake

The kids inhaled this side dish the first day I made it (along with hunks of steak), then proceeded to request it three days in a row until the leftovers were all gone. Throw in some tuna or cooked chicken and make it a full-on casserole!

Prep Time: 20 minutes

Cook Time: 30 minutes

Servings: 10

Preheat oven to 350 degrees.

Roughly chop onion, cauliflower and broccoli into bite-sized pieces. Toss together then spread vegetables evenly in a 9"x13" baking dish.

In a medium bowl add eggs, cream, salt, pepper, garlic, thyme and lemon juice. Whisk together until eggs are combined with other ingredients. Pour sauce over vegetables, gently tossing vegetables until they are coated. Sprinkle cheese on top.

Bake for 30 minutes, until edges are browning and the middle is bubbly.

Remove from oven and let rest for five minutes before serving.

OPTIONAL: Add a cup of previously cooked chopped chicken, tuna, pork, or beef to add the substance of a main dish.

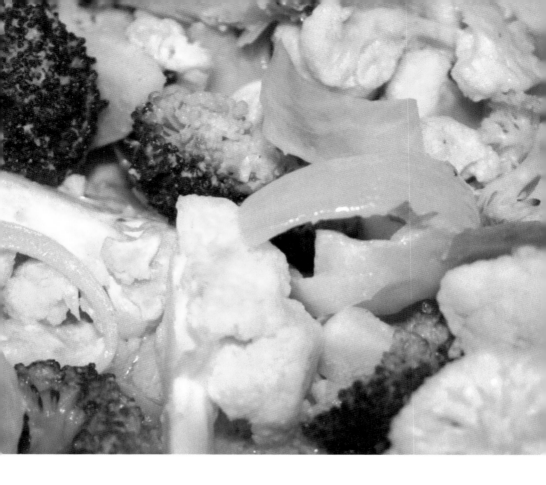

1 crown broccoli
½ head cauliflower
½ head cabbage
1 small onion
½ cup butter, melted
½ cup heavy cream
¼ cup yellow mustard
1 teaspoon garlic powder
½ teaspoon turmeric
1 teaspoon salt
Additional salt to taste

Creamy Vegetable Bake

I have found this baked vegetable dish goes really well with spicy meat. The creamy sauce and vegetable mix soothes the tongue, if you are otherwise serving it along with heat!

Prep Time: 20 minutes

Cook Time: 1 hour

Servings: 10

Preheat oven to 350 degrees.

Cut vegetables into bite-size pieces. Mix vegetables together in a 9"x13" baking dish.

In a medium bowl combine butter, cream, mustard, garlic, salt and turmeric. Whisk until well combined.

Pour sauce over vegetables and toss until coated. Cover with aluminum foil and bake for 45 minutes. Uncover and bake for an additional 15–30 minutes or more until vegetables are of preferred softness.

Serve immediately and make sure the sauce is drizzled over the top.

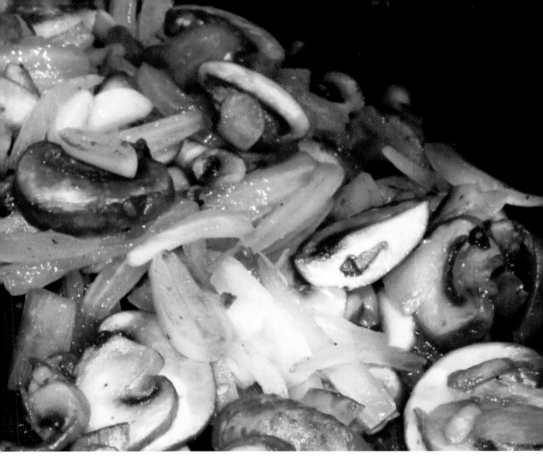

2 tablespoons butter
4 cups mini portobello or white button mushrooms,
   sliced
1 medium white onion, cut into narrow strips
4 garlic cloves, cut into quarters
¼ cup fresh, finely chopped parsley
Salt to taste

Mushroom Onion Sauté

Here is a quick side dish that works with grilled stuff, and anything that is baking in the oven and needs something on the side. I sometimes forget that sharing main dishes can overshadow the often quick and easy sides, which are not to be discounted or forgotten. I remember, back when I first began to cook on my own, I always though complicated meant better-tasting, and I was sooooo wrong!

Simple is better, but complicated is still fun! Try this. Can't go wrong.

Prep Time: 10 minutes

Cook Time: 10 minutes

Servings: 6

In medium frying pan over medium high heat, add butter. When butter is melted, add onion and garlic. Toss until coated with butter and let cook until they release water (sweat).

Lower heat to medium. Add mushrooms and parsley. Toss until well mixed and coated. Continue cooking until mushrooms soften and onions begin to brown, about eight minutes. Season with salt and cook three more minutes until salt is able to saturate vegetables.

Remove from heat and cover until ready to serve. When served with or on top of grilled meats, these vegetables soak up meat juices and complement them well.

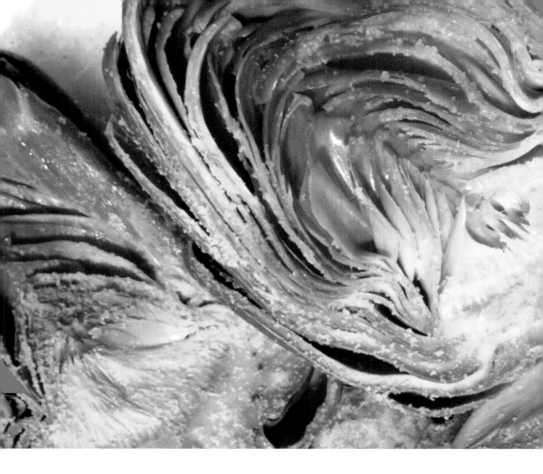

4 medium artichokes
1 cup water
¼ cup extra virgin olive oil
⅓ cup lemon juice
1 tablespoon finely chopped garlic
1 teaspoon salt
Butter
1 cup salted butter
1 teaspoon finely chopped garlic
2 tablespoons lemon juice
Salt to taste

Lemon-Infused Artichokes

To get more of the lemon and garlic flavor deeper into the artichoke I cut them in half. I don't want them to dry out, so I surround them with moisture and cover it all up. The fun thing about making these for a dinner party is watching the guests try to be dainty and tidy while eating them.

Although some places (like fancy schmancy restaurants) discard every bit of the artichoke except the heart (which can be cut into about four bites), many like dipping the meaty part of the leaves in butter and pulling it off with teeth. That would be us!

Unlike the steamed artichokes in the Appetizer section of this book, intended to be shared by a group, these halves can be served as a side dish, or at a fancier sit down dinner as individual appetizer portions.

Prep Time: 20 minutes

Cook Time: 1 hour

Servings: 8

Preheat oven to 300 degrees. In a large baking dish, add the water and about 1 tablespoon of lemon juice.

Cut the stems off the artichokes until there is only about ½ inch left, then cut them in half. Drizzle the cut side of the halves with oil and remaining lemon juice, then sprinkle with garlic and salt. Arrange halves loosely in the dish, cut side up. Cover and place in oven. Cook for about an hour until tender.

If the heart, above the stem, is not tender when gently poked with a fork, then cook them for 10 - 15 minutes longer.

While the artichokes bake, prepare the butter–in a small sauce pan over low heat add the butter, garlic and lemon juice. When butter melts stir, cover and let simmer for about one minute, then turn off heat. Add salt as desired and stir. Serve as a dipping sauce with the artichokes or drizzle it over the artichoke halves when served.

Prior to serving the artichokes, make sure to remove the hairy purple and white choke portions of the vegetable, right above the heart, and discard. Spooning it out should be easy, since it is exposed when the artichokes are cut in half.

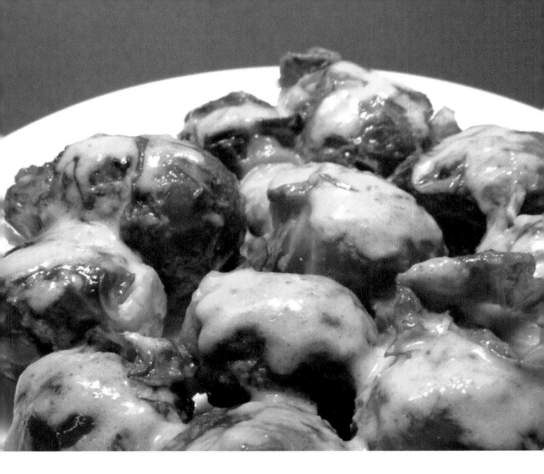

1 large stalk Brussels sprouts (about 50-60
  sprouts)
½ cup heavy cream
¼ cup butter
2 cloves garlic, crushed
½ teaspoon salt

Brussels Sprouts in Cream Sauce

Could I ignore it? Just walk by as if it were not there? Pretend it would not be loads of fun to explore? No, I was not strong enough. It drew me towards it like no other stalk. I became a stalker. A stalker of of Brussels sprout stalks. Brussels sprouts are a relative of green cabbage–high in fiber, good for you, and the sprouts grow on stalks! I usually see them in the store in bags, but sometimes they do arrive on the stalk. How fun!

My daughter was so excited about this strange thing when I got home, she could hardly wait until they were cooked.

Whenever I can, I try to show the kids where their food comes from–from pulling wild garlic, showing how vanilla pods come from orchids, to the fact that breakfast sausage comes from pigs.

I showed her the stalks and explained what the sprouts were. She immediately wanted one raw. Um, okay. I gave it to her, she took a big bite, and she LOVED IT! Chewed it up like Halloween candy! Score!

Prep Time: 5 minutes

Cook Time: 20 minutes

Servings: 10

Cut sprouts off of the stalk, leaving enough stem on each to hold the sprouts together.

In a large sauté pan with cover, melt the butter over medium heat. Add garlic and cook until you can smell the garlic aroma. Add sprouts and toss to coat them with butter. Sprinkle with salt. Cover and let cook until sprouts are softened, about ten minutes.

Lower the temperature to simmer and add the cream. Gently stir–enough to blend the cream into the sauce, but gently enough to prevent the sprouts from falling apart. Simmer covered for a few more minutes until the sauces is hot, bubbly and begins to brown, about four or five minutes. Serve immediately.

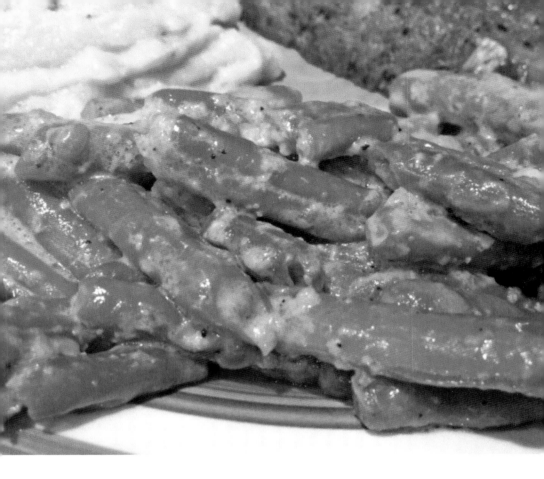

4 cups fresh green beans, steamed (or 2 cans green
   beans, drained)
¼ teaspoon ground black pepper
½ teaspoon salt
1 teaspoon garlic powder
½ teaspoon onion powder
2 tablespoons butter
¼ cup heavy whipping cream
¼ cup Worcestershire sauce
½ cup Parmesan cheese

Quick Savory Green Beans

Every once in a while I get a craving for green bean casserole. You know, the kind you usually only have as part of holiday meals? Since we are not a few days past a holiday, there is missing from the fridge a casserole dish waiting for me to empty it.

In the spirit of immediate gratification I have to act fast. These beans cook up quickly on the stovetop and are ready by the time leftover meats heat up in the oven, and wow do they hit the spot flavor-wise.

Voila! The flavor of green bean casserole without the carbohydrates and without the baking. Definitely something I am able to easily make up with our pantry staples.

Prep Time: 5 minutes

Cook Time: 20 minutes

Servings: 8

In a dry skillet over medium high heat, add the beans. Sauté until they begin to dry a bit and sear, about five minutes. Add the pepper, salt, garlic powder and onion powder. Toss and cook for another minute.

Clear a spot in the middle of the pan and add the butter, Parmesan cheese, and Worcestershire sauce. Stir into the beans as the butter melts. Cook for another five minutes.

Add the cream and simmer for five minutes, allowing the cream to heat up and sauce to thicken. Serve immediately.

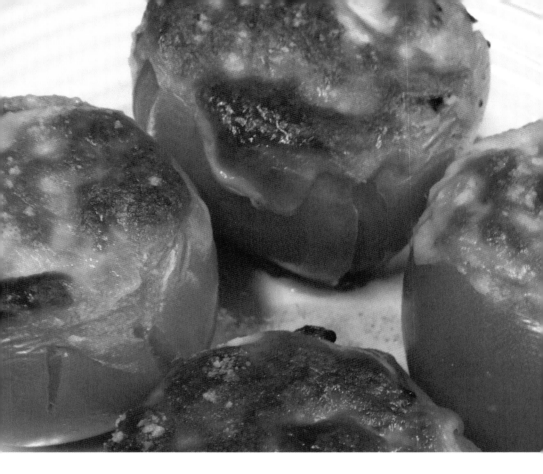

8 ripe medium size tomatoes
½ medium onion
½ green bell pepper
4 ounces white button mushrooms
2 links hot Italian sausage, cooked and
  roughly chopped
4 cloves garlic
2 tablespoons extra virgin olive oil
½ teaspoon cayenne pepper powder
½ teaspoon salt
¼ teaspoon ground black pepper
2 teaspoons hot sauce (I suggest Crystal
  or Tabasco)
1 cup mozzarella cheese
¼ cup grated Parmesan cheese
Salt and ground black pepper to taste

Prep Time: 30 minutes

Cook Time: 30 minutes

Servings: 8

Spicy Stuffed Tomatoes

We often have fresh tomatoes in our kitchen and chop them up raw as a quick side dish, but I decided this time to stuff them and bake them. The cooler weather leads me towards warm food. You can never have too many variations on vegetable dishes, can you?

I used to make these with oatmeal as filler, but since using it would conflict with eating grain free, I now replace it by adding more veggies and sausage. Works out great!

Set tomatoes on the counter so they sit on the bottoms. Cut off top portion of each tomato so the top opening is parallel to the counter, leaving them as tall as possible with a flat top. Scrape out seeds and meat core from inside of tomato. Turn tomatoes cut side down on a towel to allow extra juice to run out.

Finely chop mushrooms, onion, bell pepper and garlic. Heat oil in a medium sauté pan over medium high heat. Add garlic and onion into pan and cook about three minutes, until onions begin to sweat. Add bell pepper and mushrooms, cooking another five minutes until onions begin to brown and mushrooms release their liquid. Add cayenne pepper powder, salt, black pepper and hot sauce. Stir and simmer on low for five more minutes. Remove from heat and let cool slightly.

Preheat oven to 350 degrees.

Flip over tomatoes so cut side is up. Sprinkle the inside of each with salt and ground black pepper to taste. Drop some sausage into the bottom of each tomato, dividing it evenly among the eight tomatoes. Spoon sautéed mixture into each tomato, dividing it equally among the eight tomatoes as well.

Place stuffed tomatoes in a baking dish that allows them to fit snugly, so as to support each other while cooking. Dish size can vary due to size of tomatoes, but 9"x9" should work. Spoon ⅛ cup mozzarella cheese on the top of each tomato, pressing it down firmly so it stays on top of each.

Sprinkle Parmesan cheese on top of each tomato.

Bake for 30-35 minutes, until cheese browns and tomato skin wrinkles and begins to crack. Remove from oven and serve immediately.

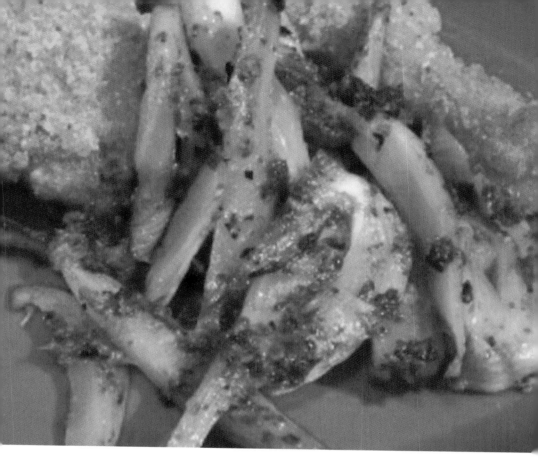

2 large fennel
2 tablespoons avocado oil
Salt and pepper to taste
½ cup olive tapenade* (see Sauce section
    for recipe)
2 tablespoons Parmesan cheese

*If you do not have prepared tapenade you can substitute
finely chopped olives. The flavor will be less intense, but
still lovely.

Fennel And Olives

I first made this when we were having some crispy oven baked chicken for dinner and thought it would be complemented by a strongly flavored side dish. The fennel, with its hint of anise, I thought would go well with some tapenade and cheese. The more subtle taste of the chicken, or any mild main dish, goes well with the powerful fennel and briny olives.

Prep Time: 10 minutes

Cook Time: 15 minutes

Servings: 8

Remove green stalks from fennel bulbs. Slice bulbs in a julienne, about eight to ten slices per bulb, depending on their size.

In a medium sauté pan over medium high heat, add the oil. When oil is hot, add the fennel. Sprinkle with salt and pepper. Toss every two minutes until fennel is browned and softening.

Add tapenade and cheese, stirring until it coats the fennel. Cover pan and lower heat to medium. Cook for another five minutes, until preferred tenderness. Remove from pan and serve immediately.

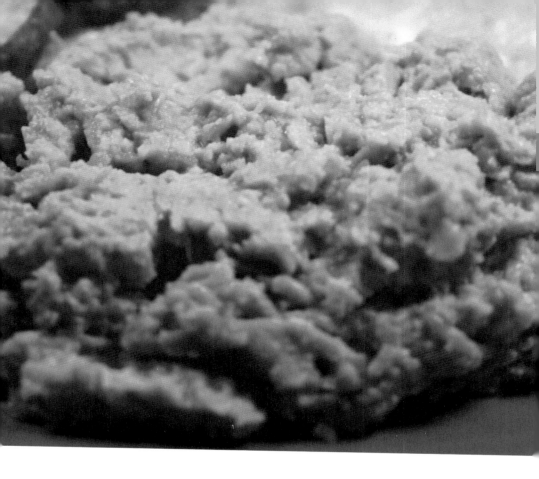

2 pounds frozen peas
½ small onion, finely diced
2 tablespoons butter
1 tablespoon fresh mint, minced leaves
  only
2 tablespoons whole milk or cream
Salt and Pepper to taste

Mushed Peas

On the first day of my first trip to Ireland I stayed up for 36 hours straight. The original plan was to sleep on the flight over the Atlantic, but a merry band of fine looking Italian men decided to have a party about five rows away, so any thoughts of peace and quiet went out the window. There are worse reasons for not sleeping. We landed in Shannon, went through customs, found our B&B, and took off in our little car to explore.

Bumping along a narrow road on the way to the Cliffs of Moher we came across a little cottage converted into a cafe. Our rumbling stomachs could be heard over the car engine, so we stopped for a bite.

It may have been the beautiful, lush green surroundings, but the fish and chips with mushed peas we ate for lunch tasted magical. Our table of two made up half the customers in the place for the entirety of our meal. It was quiet, we could see through windows in three directions, and we were slightly punchy from being awake in our 30th hour. It was a blissful break from the rushed feeling inherent to travel.

Decades later, I still recall the cup of bright peas, the subtle mint mixed in, and how amazed I was that I never thought of mushing them before. Some people call them mashed, others mushy, but I call them mushed because that is what they were called during my first encounter. Oh, and the Cliffs of Moher are quite grand and otherwise left me speechless.

Prep Time: 5 minutes

Cook Time: 10 minutes

Servings: 8

Melt butter in a pot. Add peas and onion and cook covered on low until peas and onion are tender, about eight minutes.

Add mint. Mash with a potato masher, food processor, hand blender or other macerating device you may have handy.

Add milk and stir. Season to taste with salt and pepper, but take care with quantities, because a little goes a long way with mushed peas. Serve warm with fish, shrimp, or pork.

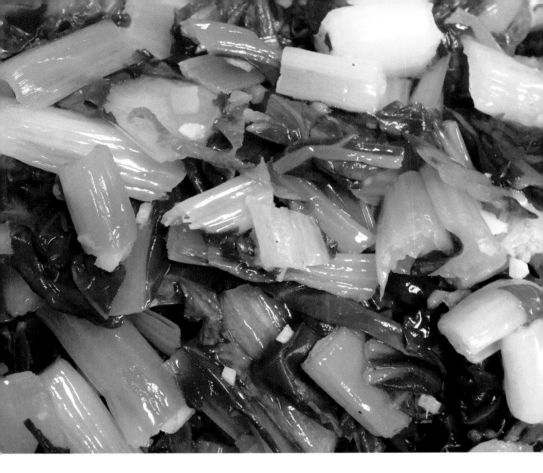

2 - 4 bunches bok choy, well rinsed (to equal to
  approximately 8 cups raw chopped)
1 tablespoon coconut oil
1 tablespoon ginger, peeled and finely minced, or
  1 ½ teaspoons ground ginger
2 cloves garlic, finely minced
1 teaspoon salt
½ teaspoon ground black pepper

Bright Bok Choy

Eating bok choy keeps with the trend in our house of eating green, leafy vegetables as often as possible. I like mustard greens and turnip greens and collard greens and spinach, but any variety is welcome in my world. Especially when it is fun to say—bok choy, bok choy, bok choy, bok choy…

Prep Time: 10 minutes
Cook Time: 15 minutes

Servings: 8

Thoroughly rinse sand and soil from bok choy. Chop green leaves off from white stems. Loosely chop green tops. Chop white stems to bite-sized pieces.

Add oil to wok or large frying pan over medium high heat. When oil is hot, add ginger and garlic. Cook until it begins to brown.

Add chopped white stems. Cook stems for about five minutes, tossing regularly.

Add green tops and sprinkle with salt and pepper. Toss mixture until greens are wilted, 3-5 minutes. Season with additional salt to taste. Remove to serving bowl and serve immediately.

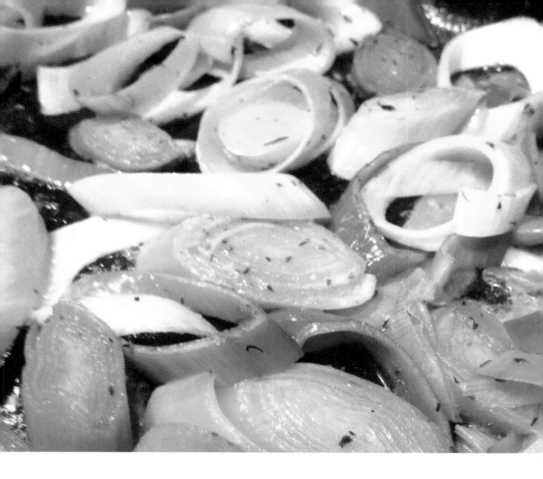

2 leeks
½ cup butter
1 tablespoon dried thyme leaves
½ teaspoon salt
⅛ teaspoon ground black pepper

Buttered Leeks

I really like how much leeks brighten up a plate when I use the whole leek. So many recipes involving leeks focus on the white part and pretend the green parts don't exist. Where do they think the white parts would be without the green? Never disrespect the green.

Prep Time: 5 minutes

Cook Time: 25 minutes

Servings: 8

Trim off dried leek tips of green portion and roots of white portion. Slice entirety of leek (yes, green and white sections) in thin diagonal pieces.

In a large frying pan, over medium high heat, melt the butter. Add thyme, salt and pepper. Stir. Add leeks.

Toss until butter mixture coats all pieces of leek. Continue stirring for five minutes.

Reduce heat to low and cover pan, cooking for an additional 15 minutes. Leeks should still be bright green but tender. Remove top and salt more to taste.

Stir again and serve immediately.

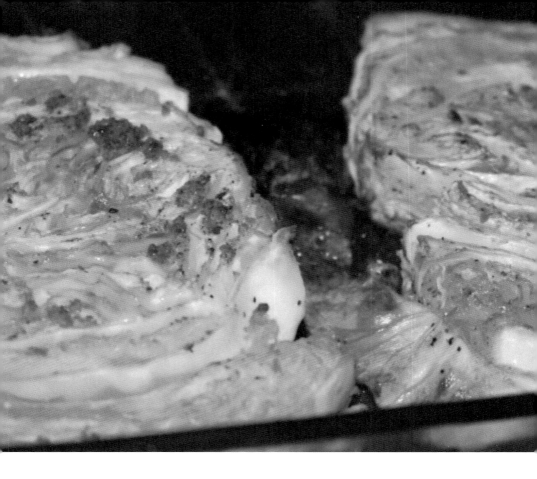

1 small head green cabbage
1 teaspoon chopped fresh garlic
1 teaspoon chopped fresh ginger
½ teaspoon ground nutmeg
2 tablespoons olive oil
2 tablespoons butter (use more olive oil instead for
  dairy free)
Salt and Pepper to taste

Roasted Cabbage

Roasting cabbage in the oven brings out the flavor without it getting soggy. It is easy to cook up while something is finishing up on the grill or crock pot/pressure cooker. Enjoy!

Prep Time: 10 minutes

Cook Time: 1 hour

Servings: 8

Preheat oven to 375F.

Cut the cabbage head in half, leaving the stem attached. Out of each half cut a 1" thick slice. Trim some of the stem out of the slices, but leave enough to help hold the leaves together. Set aside the outer, domed slices for another use, like coleslaw or sauté.

In a large rectangular baking dish, or sheet pan, drizzle 1 tablespoon of the oil. Sprinkle the garlic and ginger, as well as some salt and pepper, over the oil in a shape approximate to the circumference of the cabbage slices.

Place the slices on the pan, gently pressing down so the spices are pushed into the cabbage. Place a pat of butter on top of the slices, along with more salt and pepper.

Bake for about 30 minutes, then flip the slices. Bake for 30 more minutes, or until cabbage is softened to preferred tenderness. Serve immediately.

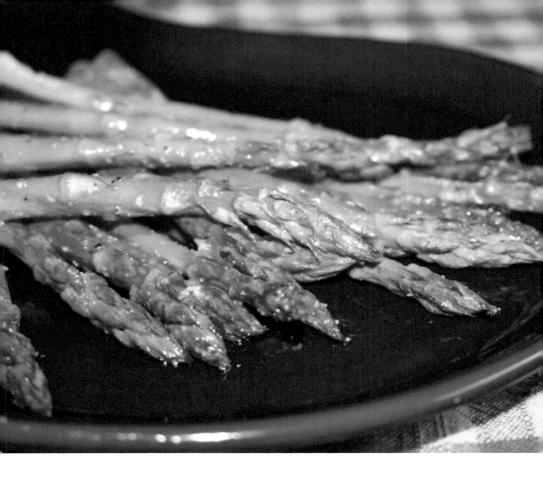

1 large bunch raw asparagus
2 tablespoons olive oil
1 tablespoon lime juice
½ cup chopped pecans or almonds (optional)
2 cloves garlic, diced
2 tablespoons Parmesan cheese
Salt and ground black pepper to taste

Roasted Asparagus

For a long time I had so much trouble cooking asparagus well. I either undercooked it or overcooked it into a green mush. Now it comes out perfectly every time–the thick ends are soft enough to eat and the delicate tips still have substance. The roasting really brings out the flavor of the asparagus while making it tender to eat, hot or cold.

I have often taken leftovers on picnics or in cold lunches and it works just as well as if it is right out of the oven. So simple and so scrumptious! Thanks to my longtime friend Karla for showing me how to make it at a dinner party in Denver!

Prep Time: 15 minutes

Cook Time: 35 minutes

Servings: 6

Heat oven to 350F. Rinse asparagus and remove the thick, tough ends. You can do this in any of three different ways:
1. Cut the bottom 1-2 inches off with a knife, or
2. Bend the stalk until it naturally breaks where the tough section begins, or
3. For thicker stalks, use a vegetable peeler to gently peel off thick outer skin from the bottom half of the stalk; no need to chop off any length except the very end.

Line a cookie sheet with aluminum foil. Lay asparagus on foil, alternating thick and thin ends. Make sure the stalks alternate the direction of the tip, so they can cook evenly.

Sprinkle asparagus with olive oil and lime juice, followed by garlic, salt, pepper and nuts. Place in oven on the middle rack for 20-30 minutes, until tender.

Sprinkle with Parmesan cheese and return to oven, cooking for about five more minutes until cheese is soft. Serve immediately.

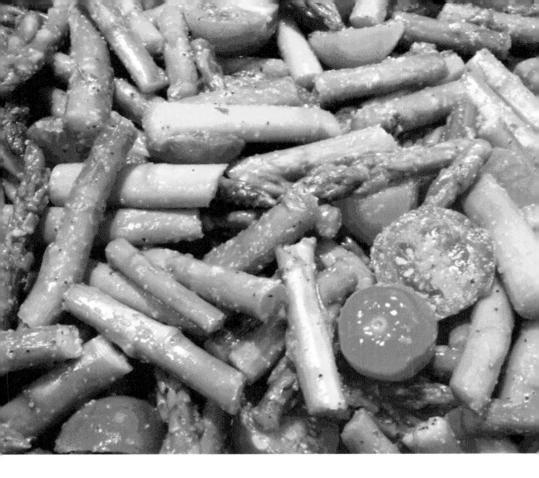

2 tablespoons extra virgin olive oil
2 bunches asparagus
2 cups small tomatoes or cherry tomatoes
1 teaspoon garlic powder
Salt and pepper to taste

Asparagus Tomato Sauté

When preparing this dish, the tomatoes wilted and balanced the enjoyable bitterness of the asparagus. Goes great with roasted or grilled meats and can be done easily on the stovetop.

Prep Time: 10 minutes

Cook Time: 15 minutes

Servings: 12

Slice off the last one to two inches of the the thick ends of the asparagus and discard. Cut the remaining asparagus stalks into bite-sized pieces, about one inch each. Slice tomatoes in half or thirds, making sure they are bite-sized. If using small cherry tomatoes they can be left whole.

Heat oil in a large sauté pan over medium high heat. Add asparagus and stir until slightly softened, about five minutes. Add tomatoes and stir. Sprinkle with garlic, salt and pepper to taste. Stir so as to spread out the spices.

Turn down heat, cover and simmer, cooking for about five more minutes, until the asparagus is softened as desired. Turn off heat and leave covered until time to serve.

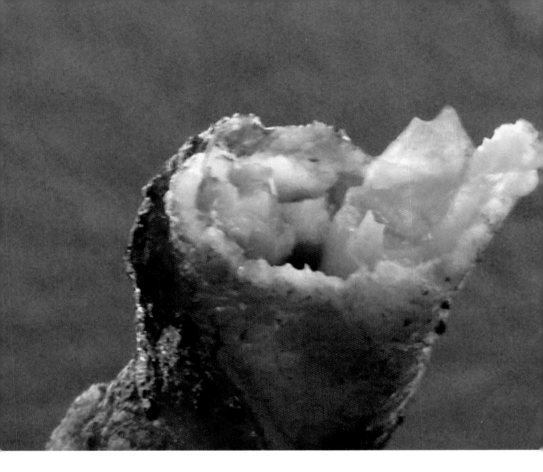

1 pound asparagus spears, tough ends removed
1 pound sliced bacon, room temperature

Bacon-Wrapped Asparagus

Although easy to serve as a side dish daintily cut up alongside a steak, we usually scarf them down with our fingers. I also cook them up on a pan in the oven.

Prep Time: 10 minutes

Cook Time: 10 minutes

Servings: 8

Combine asparagus spears in multiple bundles so each one does not exceed ½ inch diameter, usually one or two spears.

Wrap a strip of bacon around each bundle at a diagonal, so most of the asparagus is covered. The bacon will overlap on one end, which will help hold the bacon on the asparagus.

Cooking approaches:

1. Grill bundles over a charcoal fire of medium to high heat until bacon is crisp. This can be done directly on the grates, or by using a grilling basket. Remove and let cool until safe to eat, or
2. Heat the broiler to medium and place on broiling pan. If your oven does not have more than one broiler setting you can lower the rack to better control the cooking speed. When top side is crisp (three to five minutes), turn over to crisp on underside. Remove from broiler and let cool.

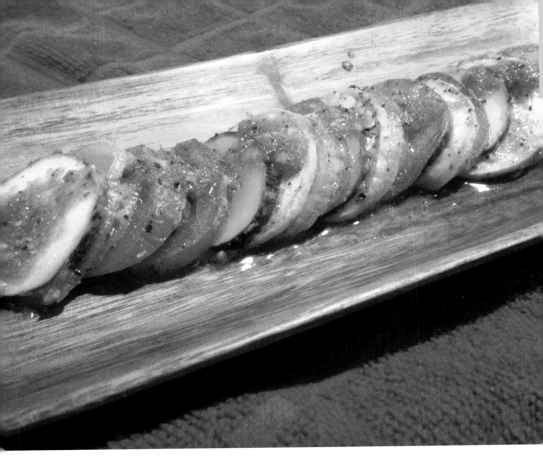

1 medium zucchini
1 medium yellow squash
2 medium onions
3 large Roma tomatoes
2 cups diced tomatoes
2 cloves garlic, crushed
1 tablespoon dried oregano leaves
1 tablespoon dried parsley leaves
½ teaspoon salt
¼ teaspoon ground black pepper

Ratatouille

I think this is ratatouille, but some people may find it lacking. What I love about it is the combination of flavors I get from the alternating, thinly sliced vegetables in a single bite.

I like bell peppers in general, which are usually included in this dish, but I don't like the taste and texture they add to the other veggies used here, so I left them out. Look at me being a ratatouille rebel!

A neat thing about this recipe is it can be doubled and tripled easily by adding more sliced vegetables and a larger pan. It also makes for a lovely presentation in a serving dish or on your plate.

Prep Time: 30 minutes

Cook Time: 50 minutes

Servings: 8

In a medium pot over medium heat add the diced tomatoes, garlic, oregano, parsley, salt and pepper. Simmer for about ten minutes, until heated through and bubbly, while you prepare other ingredients. Remove from heat to let cool.

Preheat oven to 375 degrees.

While sauce simmers, prepare the zucchini, yellow squash, onion and Roma tomatoes by slicing them thinly, about ⅛ inch thick. Removing seeds from tomatoes is optional–if they have a lot of seeds it may be a good idea. Sprinkle slices with salt and pepper.

Using a stand or stick blender purée the sauce until smooth.

In a loaf pan, pour a thin layer of tomato sauce (you will probably have leftover sauce). Alternate the slices of zucchini, yellow squash, tomatoes and onion, placing them in two long rows in the pan.

Bake for 30 minutes, cover pan with foil and bake for an additional 15 minutes.

Remove from oven and let sit for 5 minutes before serving.

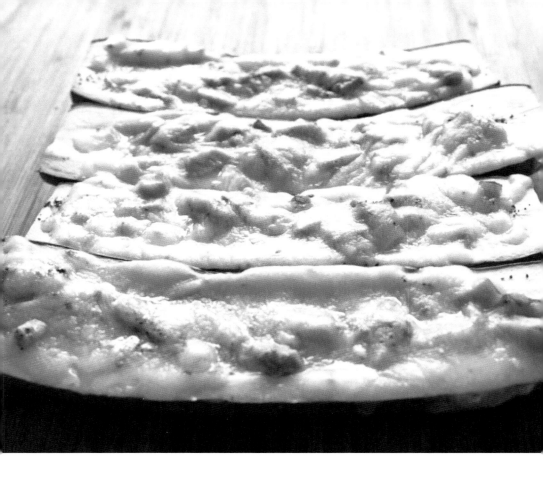

2 medium zucchini
4 small garlic cloves
1 cup diced prosciutto or cured ham
1 cup shredded Monterey Jack cheese
Salt and pepper to taste

Stuffed Courgettes

My husband is not a zucchini lover. Yellow squash? Yes. Acorn squash? Yes. Zucchini? Well, um, I guess…I figured if I topped it with meat and cheese it might work. It pretty much did.

I know. I rule. I enjoy making them with a variety of stuffings, but my favorite is the prosciutto and Monterey Jack.

Prep Time: 15 minutes

Cook Time: 30 minutes

Servings: 4

Slice ends off zucchini, then cut them in half lengthwise. With a small spoon, gently carve out the seedy belly of the halves, stopping about ½ inch from the ends, making a groove down the middle. Sprinkle each half with salt and pepper.

Slice garlic cloves into slivers and spread a clove in each half. Divide prosciutto among the halves, then top with cheese.

Place zucchini in a 9"x9" or 9"x11" baking dish, leaving a little space between them. Bake for about 30 minutes, depending on the size of the zucchini, until tender and cheese begins to brown.

Serve immediately.

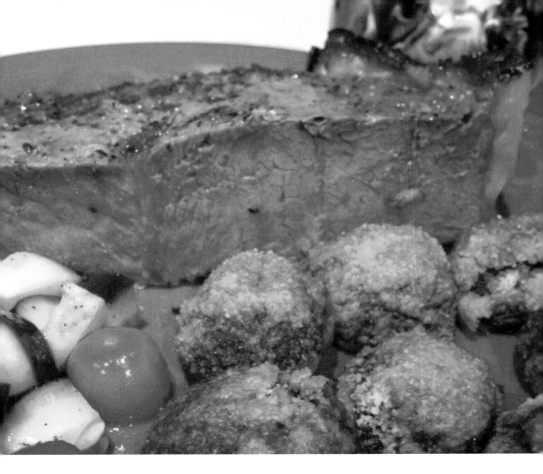

18 mini portobello or white button mushrooms
½ cup dry red wine
¼ cup lemon juice
2 teaspoons garlic powder
1½ teaspoon salt
1 tablespoon dehydrated chopped onion or 1
   teaspoon onion powder
1 cup finely grated Parmesan cheese, further
   pureed to powder in a food processor
½ cup almond flour

Baked Parmesan Mush-rooms

There is no mistaking the mushroom-ness of this side dish. It went well with some ribeye steaks we smoked up for a very satisfying dinner.

Prep Time: 20 minutes (plus 2 hours marinating)

Cook Time: 30 minutes

Servings: 6

Trim mushroom stems until they are flush with the bottom of the cap. In a shallow dish or resealable bag add the marinade ingredients–wine, lemon juice, 1 teaspoon garlic powder, 1 teaspoon salt and onion. Stir until salt dissolves.

Add mushrooms and toss in marinade until they are all coated. Leave mushrooms to marinate at room temperature for about two hours.

Preheat oven to 400 degrees.

Remove mushrooms from marinade and pat dry with towels.

In a medium bowl, combine Parmesan cheese, almond flour, 1 teaspoon garlic powder and ½ teaspoon salt. Stir dry mixture until combined.

One at a time, coat each mushroom with the dry mixture–it should stick well to the wet mushrooms. Place each mushroom stem-side down on a shallow baking sheet, evenly spaced.

Bake for 20-25 minutes, until mushrooms shrink a bit and coating begins to brown. Remove from oven and let sit for about five minutes before serving.

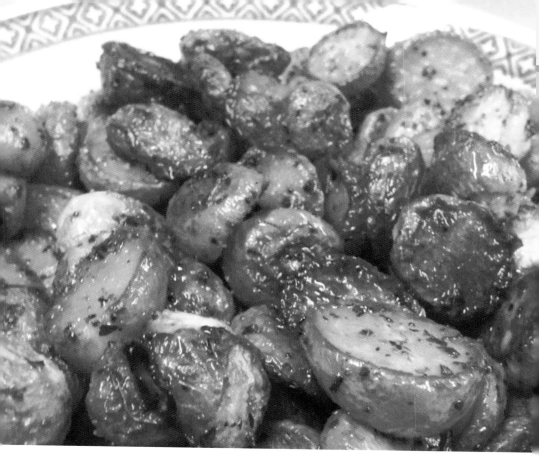

4 cups small red radishes, chopped into halves
3 tablespoons extra virgin olive oil
2 teaspoons salt
2 teaspoons granulated garlic powder
1 teaspoon dried parsley leaves
2 teaspoons dried oregano leaves

Roasted Radishes

Roasted radishes can easily be mistaken for roasted new potatoes or turnips. These guys are like vegetable candy. The radishes remind me of turnips, but much more tender and sweet from the start.

Radishes are ecstatic raw with a peppery bite to them. The great thing about radishes is that they are tender from the beginning, and only get more tender if cooked. They can be lightly roasted until just heated through, or if they are roasted a bit more, you allow for a bit of caramelizing. I did the longer cooking time here to maximize the caramelizing. They go great with anything you would serve with fried or baked potatoes.

Prep Time: 10 minutes

Cook Time: 1 hour

Servings: 8

Preheat oven to 350 degrees.

In a large bowl, combine the oil, salt, garlic, parsley and oregano. Add the radishes and toss until coated.

Spread radishes evenly on foil lined shallow baking pan. Bake for 30 minutes.

Remove from oven and toss, then return to oven for 30 minutes.

Remove from oven again and serve immediately.

POULTRY

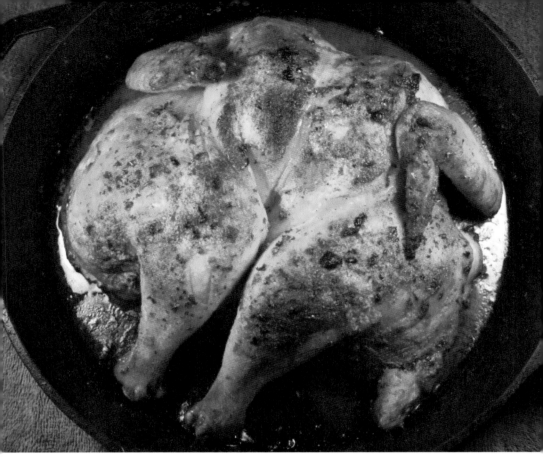

1 whole chicken, 4-5 pounds
2 tablespoons butter, room
  temperature
1 large lime
1 teaspoon salt
1 teaspoon pepper
2 teaspoons chopped garlic
1 teaspoon ground cumin
1 teaspoon onion powder
1 tablespoon chopped parsley
½ teaspoon ground sage
1 teaspoon ground thyme

Spatchcocked Chicken

To all those who have trouble cooking a roast chicken, please continue reading, for I have your solution right here. To everyone who thinks they have made a good roast chicken, you should also keep reading, because you may be wrong. Being able to roast a chicken is a good skill to have, but when you find a big one at the store there is always the challenge of getting the meat evenly cooked, considering the meat is not evenly distributed around the cavity.

One solution is sticking it on a full, open soda can and letting the soda keep it moist while standing on end and cooking. The can method works, but to me the meat gets an odd flavor. It might have been the fact I don't much like sugary sodas, or the chemicals on the can labeling, but it just tastes odd.

Splitting a chicken in half and cooking it in an iron skillet results in an amazingly moist, flavorful chicken. Since the bird is laid down almost flat the meat cooks evenly. The dark meat gets cooked instead of running red, and the white meat does not overcook for the sake of the dark meat. It also maximizes exposure of the skin for crispiness.

The first time I used the spatchcocked method, I did not expect much difference from when I roasted with the bird whole. When we started eating it, not only were the herbs and spices more evenly distributed in the meat, but taking the bird apart and carving it up was easier, because it was flat and easier to manipulate.

Prep Time: 20 minutes

Cook Time: 1 hour

Servings: 8

Preheat oven to 375 degrees.

Place chicken on a cutting surface breast side down. Using a knife cut skin and meat down to the bone, following the spine. With a sturdy pair of scissors cut right along both sides of the spine to remove it. Turn chicken over and press down in the middle between the wings until the wishbone breaks and the chicken lays down almost flat. Take care not to push it completely flat to the point the ribs break—that is too far.

Squeeze lime juice onto both sides of the chicken. Also gently pull skin away from the meat in a few places and place some of the lime meat between the skin and meat. If you have fresh herbs you can slide a sprig or two of parsley, sage or thyme under the skin to add some extra flavor. Sprinkle salt and pepper on the bottom (formerly the cavity/inside) of the chicken.

Place chicken in large iron skillet, skin side up. Get your hands dirty by spreading the butter all over the skin side of the chicken, including crevasses, until it is all gone. Sprinkle salt, pepper and herbs all over butter.

Cover with foil and put chicken in oven and cook for about an hour, removing the foil after about 30 minutes. The chicken is done when a thermometer reads 160 degrees and juices run clear.

Remove from oven and let rest for about ten minutes before serving.

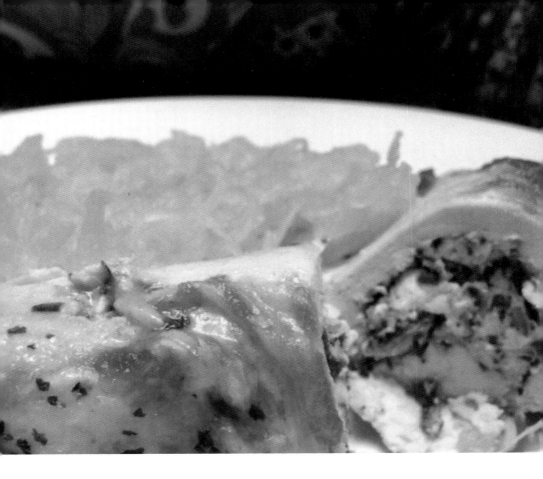

6 boneless chicken breasts
2 cups baby spinach leaves
1½ cup crumbled feta cheese
6 pieces bacon, cooked crisp
   and crumbled
1 teaspoon dried basil leaves
2 cups mozzarella, shredded
½ cup tomato sauce
1½ cups diced tomatoes
1 teaspoon garlic powder
1 teaspoon onion powder
Salt and pepper to taste

Prep Time: 30 minutes

Cook Time: 45 minutes

Servings: 6

Rolled Chicken Breasts

Besides the satisfaction of pounding flesh into oblivion, the balance of flavors is supreme with these rolls, combining the mildness of white chicken meat and kick of the stuffing.

Since the chicken was thin, the cooking time was kept short and the dish was moist, in a good way. Never hesitate to pound the meat just a little bit more, for it won't hurt the chicken, and it can't help but release anything lingering and seething in you.

I almost called this recipe 'stuffed', but since I did such a good job of pounding, the 'rolled' version of the name seemed appropriate. I served the rolls with some veggies and voila! Dinner!

Preheat oven to 350 degrees.

Pound chicken breasts with kitchen mallet until no thicker than ¼ inch.

Chop spinach finely. Combine it with the crumble bacon, feta and basil in medium bowl.

Season both sides of chicken with salt and pepper. Lay a breast flat on your work surface with the longest section going left to right. Place ¼ to ⅓ cup (divided equally among the breasts) of filling in the middle of the flat meat.

Starting from the left or right carefully roll the breast until it overlaps with the chicken on the opposite side of the filling. Place stuffed breast in a 9"x9" (snugly) or 10"x10" (close but not so snug).

Repeat with the other five breasts and place them in the dish.

Cover and place in preheated oven. Bake for about 20 minutes.

While chicken is baking combine tomatoes, tomato sauce, garlic powder and onion powder in a medium sauce pan over medium high heat. When the mixture begins to bubble turn the heat down and summer uncovered for about 15 minutes. Add salt to sauce if needed.

After chicken cooks for 20 minutes remove it from the oven. Sprinkle half the cheese on the chicken, top with the tomato sauce and then the rest of the cheese. Return the pan to the oven uncovered and cook for 15 - 20 more minutes, until the edges begin to brown.

Remove from oven and let sit for five minutes before serving.

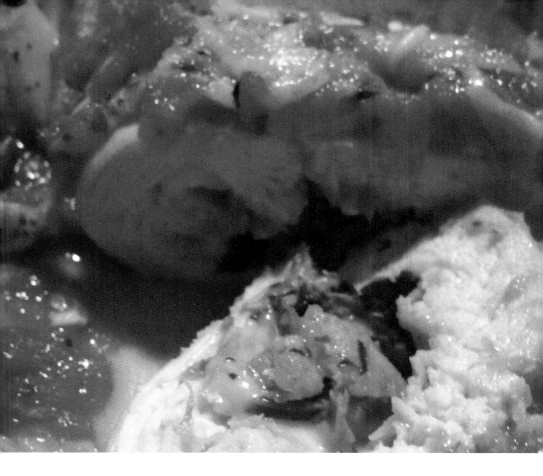

3 ½ cups diced tomatoes (if using canned, include liquid)
1 cup tomato sauce
3 garlic cloves, chopped
1 small bunch fresh parsley, stems removed
3 sprigs fresh oregano, stems removed
8-10 fresh basil leaves
1 teaspoon ground cumin
½ teaspoon ground black pepper
1 teaspoon salt
4 cups fresh spinach
2 cups (or 2 14-ounce cans) marinated artichoke hearts, drained
½ medium yellow onion, finely diced
1 tablespoon lemon juice
6 boneless skinless chicken breasts
12 slices thin deli ham
4 cups grated cheddar cheese
Salt and pepper to taste

Susan's Stuffed Chicken Breasts

Whenever my friends have news, good or bad, I want to cook for them. For good news it is a celebration! For bad news, it is my version of giving comfort. It is born from a habit started long ago with my family. We always celebrated or mourned surrounded by our people over a table full of food. One of my oldest and dearest friends came over with news one night and cooking was definitely a necessity.

She loved it when I made Rolled Chicken Breasts before, so I followed their fowl lead and came up with another rolled beauty. These chicken breasts came out much less dainty and heartily filled us up. Definitely appropriate for the occasion, since my friend has some ass kicking to do in the near future.

Prep Time: 45 minutes (including sauce)

Cook Time: 45 minutes (plus cooling)

Servings: 6

In a medium sauce pot over medium heat add the diced tomatoes, tomato sauce and garlic. Roughly chop the parsley, oregano and basil leaves. Add all the herbs except about 2 tablespoons to the sauce. Set aside the extra herbs for the top of the dish. When the sauce begins to steam, lower heat let simmer uncovered for about 30 minutes then remove from heat.

While sauce is simmering prepare the chicken and stuffing. Finely chop the spinach and artichoke hearts. In a medium bowl combine the artichoke hearts, spinach, onion and lemon juice. Toss until combined. Add salt and pepper to taste. Set aside.

Spread a piece of wax or parchment paper on the counter, at least twice the size of a single chicken breast. Place a breast in the middle of the paper. Cover the breast with a second piece of paper. With the flat side of a tenderizer mallet (or a regular mallet covered in cling wrap), gently pound the breast, starting from the center and moving towards the edges, until it is ¼ inch to ⅓ inch thick. Repeat with all the breasts, changing out the paper as needed. Generously season each breast on both sides with salt and pepper.

Preheat oven to 350 degrees.

To stuff the chicken clear a work surface. Position nearby a 9"×13" inch baking dish. Spread a thin layer of tomato sauce on the bottom of the dish. Place a single breast in front of you on your work surface lengthwise. Use two pieces of ham to cover the surface of the breast as much as possible. Sprinkle ⅓ cup of grated cheese on top of the ham. Spoon 1/6 of the spinach artichoke mixture in a row from top to bottom on one side of the breast. Starting on the side nearest the mixture begin rolling the breast, making sure the left and right ends overlap at least once at the end of the roll. Place the roll seam down in the baking dish. Repeat with the remaining breasts.

Pour tomato sauce over chicken rolls, leaving ¼ inch from the top edge clear of sauce so there is room for it to bubble up to the dish edges. You may have leftover sauce, depending on the size of the chicken breasts. Sprinkle remaining grated cheese and chopped herbs on top of the sauce.

Bake for 45 minutes until chicken is thoroughly cooked, to at least 160 degrees. Remove from oven and let sit for ten minutes before serving.

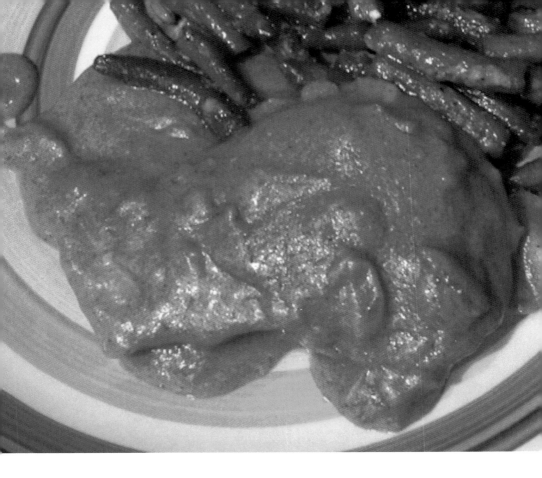

2 tablespoons butter or oil
8 skinless boneless chicken thighs
½ white onion finely chopped
4 cloves garlic, finely chopped
½ cup natural peanut butter
15 ounces tomato sauce
½ cup lemon juice
2 tablespoons ground turmeric
2 teaspoons ground ginger
1 teaspoon ground cinnamon
1 tablespoon cayenne pepper
1 teaspoon salt
1 teaspoon ground black pepper
8 ounces full fat coconut milk

Red Chicken

This recipe represents my first gander at being inspired by a Northern Indian dish called Butter Chicken. The final product is far from accurate with the name, so I am not even trying to use butter in the title. I have also used this sauce for Red Eggs in an earlier section of this book.

Prep Time: 10 minutes

Cook Time: 40 minutes

Servings: 8

In medium sauté pan over medium high heat melt butter. Add chicken and partially cook, about five minutes, flipping half way through. Remove chicken from pan and set aside.

Add to the the pan juices the onion and garlic, cooking until browning begins. Add remaining ingredients except for coconut milk. Stir until all ingredients are combined, turning down heat to medium low, and simmering for about ten minutes until hot and bubbly.

Add coconut milk and stir again until combined.

Add chicken and simmer until cooked through, about ten more minutes.

Serve immediately. Leftover sauce can be used to poach eggs, to make shakshuka, for Red Eggs.

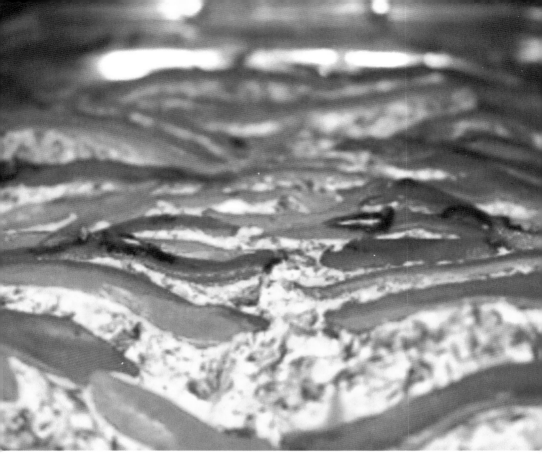

8 chicken thighs, skin on

3 cups fresh spinach, roughly chopped (or 1 9-ounce pkg frozen, thawed and excess water squeezed out)

1 tablespoon extra virgin olive oil

6 cloves garlic, crushed

8 ounces cream cheese

4 ounces goat cheese

6 ounces sour cream

½ teaspoon salt

2 tablespoons lime juice

3 roasted red peppers, jarred or fresh roasted, with skin removed

Salt and pepper to taste

Baked Spinach Pepper Chicken

This stuff is pretty rich, and I spooned up every bit of the sauce, and slurped it up like soup when the chicken was long gone. That is all.

Prep Time: 20 minutes

Cook Time: 50 minutes

Servings: 8

Preheat oven to 375 degrees.

Lightly salt and pepper chicken thighs after trimming off excess fat and skin. Leave enough skin on to cover the top of the chicken thigh meat. If you prefer, remove all the skin. I suggest leaving it on to release fat that helps keep the the chicken juicy.

Place one layer of chicken in 9"x13" inch baking dish.

Slice red peppers into thin strips, no more than ¼ inch width and set aside.

In a medium pot over medium high heat, add olive oil. When oil is hot add garlic. When garlic begins to brown add spinach. Lower heat to medium low. When spinach is hot and wilted, add cream cheese, goat cheese, sour cream, salt and juice. Stir until cheeses are melted and combined with spinach and garlic.

Spread cheese and spinach mixture over chicken. Lay slices of red pepper over cheese mixture so they are evenly distributed. Cover pan with aluminum foil. Bake for 20 minutes.

Remove foil and cook for 20 - 25 more minutes until peppers are dried out a bit, cheese is bubbly, and the chicken is cooked through.

Let sit for about five minutes before serving.

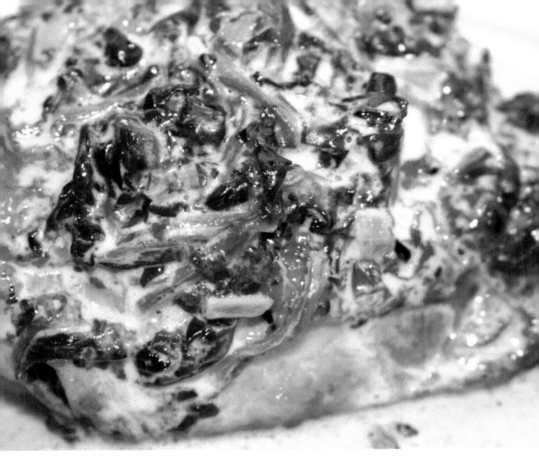

8 bone-in chicken thighs, skin attached
1 tablespoon butter
1 cup heavy cream
5 ounces frozen spinach, thawed and excess water
  squeezed out
½ small white onion, chopped
3 garlic cloves, diced
¾ cup shredded Parmesan cheese
Salt and pepper to taste

Creamy Spinach Chicken

In my quest to always find a new way to prepare chicken I came up with this lovely, rich dish that incorporates my favorite vegetable– spinach!

Prep Time: 15 minutes

Cook Time: 30 minutes

Servings: 8

On medium high heat sear chicken thighs on both sides, making sure the skin gets crispy, about 10 minutes total, most of the time spent with skin side down.

While the chicken cooks, melt butter over medium heat in a sauce pan. Add onion and garlic and cook until translucent. Add spinach and stir until heated through. Add cream and turn down heat, but bring sauce to a simmer and let cook for about five minutes. Add cheese and stir until melted and combined.

When chicken is seared, remove from pan and discard juices*. Return chicken to pan and pour sauce over chicken. Simmer covered over low heat until chicken is cooked through, about five more minutes. Serve immediately and make sure you drizzle sauce over every piece.

*The juices can be left in the pan, but will dilute and thin the sauce more than ideal.

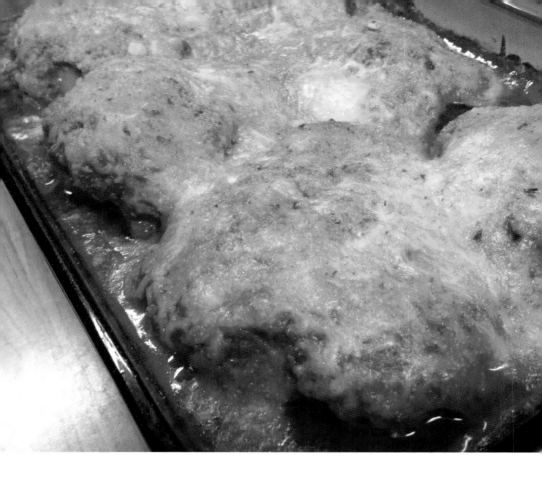

2 pounds fresh tomatoes (about 4 cups diced)
3 garlic cloves, crushed
½ medium yellow or white onion, chopped
1 cup fresh basil leaves
¼ cup fresh oregano leaves
1 cup fresh parsley leaves
4 cups fresh, raw spinach
2 teaspoons salt
1 teaspoon ground black pepper
⅓ cup heavy whipping cream
8–10 chicken thighs, bone in and skin on
Salt and pepper, to season chicken
1 cup finely grated Parmesan cheese
2 cups grated mozzarella cheese
¼ cup finely chopped mixed fresh herbs (optional)

Prep Time: 1 hour (includes sauce cook time)

Cook Time: 55 minutes

Servings: 8

Baked Garden Chicken

Much of what you need for garden chicken can come from your garden, or your neighbor's garden, or even your local farmers' market vendor gardens…the first time I made it the herbs came from my brother's garden. The dish is full of summer and the sauce, which can be made in advance of baking the chicken, is addictive. You have been warned.

Roughly chop tomatoes and place in large sauce pan uncovered over medium high heat. Add onion, garlic, basil, oregano and parsley. When mixture is bubbly reduce heat to medium and continue cooking uncovered for 30–45 minutes, until liquid from tomatoes is released and reduced by about half.

Add the spinach, salt, and pepper, stirring until the spinach wilts and mixes with the tomatoes. Let simmer for ten more minutes. Remove pan from heat. With an immersion blender (or carefully pour the hot stuff into a stand blender) purée the sauce until tomatoes, spinach and herbs are blended into a smooth sauce. Add the heavy whipping cream to the tomato sauce and simmer for five more minutes until it is reheated. Remove from heat.

Preheat oven to 350 degrees.

Spread a thin layer of tomato sauce on the bottom of a 9"x13" baking dish. Season chicken on both sides with salt and pepper, then place them in the dish. Sprinkle half the Parmesan cheese over the chicken thighs.

Pour tomato spinach sauce over chicken, making sure it is covered. Sprinkle mozzarella cheese and optional chopped herbs over chicken, followed by the rest of the Parmesan cheese.

Place in oven and bake for 30 minutes. Cheeses should begin to brown. Cover dish loosely with aluminum foil (to prevent cheese from getting too brown) and bake for 15 more minutes.

Remove from oven and let sit for 10 minutes before serving.

When serving, gently lift the chicken out of the dish, trying not to disturb the sauce and cheese that have settled on top of each thigh–as the dish cooked the tomato solids settled on top of the chicken with the cheeses and the juices ran down, so serving with the 'topping' intact makes for a pretty presentation.

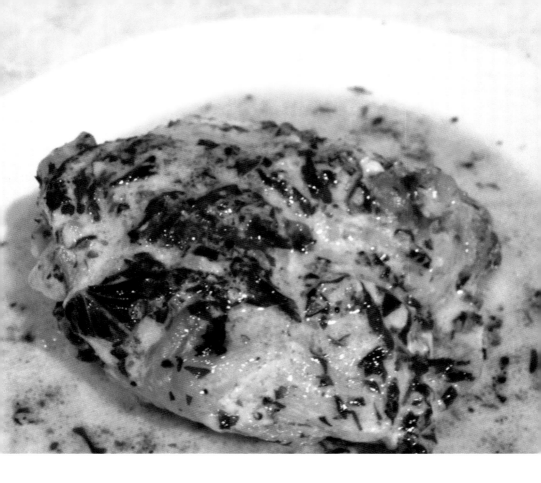

8 bone in chicken thighs, skin on
¼ cup butter
¾ – 1 cup heavy whipping cream
1 cup fresh parsley
1 cup fresh cilantro
½ cup fresh basil
3 cloves garlic, chopped
Salt and pepper to taste

Herbilicious Pan Chicken

It is so herby and so delicious it must be herbilicious! And chicken to boot!

Prep Time: 10 minutes

Cook Time: 25 minutes

Servings: 8

Season chicken thighs with salt and pepper.

In a large frying pan over medium high heat, place all thighs in the dry plan, skin side down. Cook until skin begins to brown, about eight minutes. Turn thighs and cook for five more minutes.

While chicken cooks, roll the parsley, cilantro and basil together and slice them up, then finish with a rough chop.

Add butter to pan, let it melt, then flip thighs so they are all coated with butter.

Add herbs and garlic, again turning the thighs so they are coated. Cover pan and cook for ten more minutes, until juices from chicken run clear.

Add cream and stir thighs until cream mixes with juices and herbs. Lower heat and let simmer until cream is heated and chicken is cooked completely, about five more minutes.

Serve immediately.

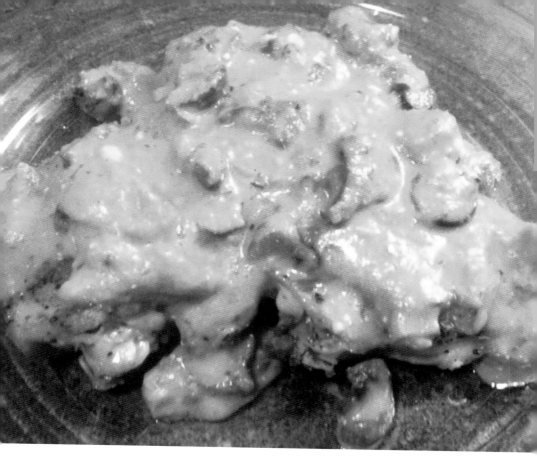

1 tablespoon butter
8 ounces white button mushrooms, roughly chopped
½ teaspoon salt
¼ white or yellow onion, finely diced
4 ounces chopped black olives
3 cloves garlic, minced
1 - 14.5 ounce can fire roasted diced tomatoes
1 - 15 ounce can tomato sauce
1 tablespoon dried parsley leaves
2 teaspoons dried oregano leaves
8 bone in chicken thighs, skin trimmed, but some left
  on meat
4 ounces cream cheese
1 tablespoon hot sauce

Non Vodka Chicken

The thing about vodka sauce is not necessarily the vodka, but what it does to the flavor of the tomatoes. The vodka, when used, actually soaks into the tomatoes and enhances their flavor for a further tart tanginess. The alcohol itself evaporates. If you have had the sauce before you know what I mean. If not, then imagine a mild bloody mary—a skidge of pepper and hot sauce—not too ferocious, but an extra bite beyond plain tomato. This recipe totally did the job taking care of my craving.

Prep Time: 10 minutes

Cook Time: 1 hour (including sauce)

Servings: 8

In a medium sauce pan over medium high heat, melt butter. Add mushrooms, salt, olives and garlic. sauté for about five minutes until mushrooms and garlic soften and butter browns a bit.

Add tomatoes and tomato sauce, parsley and oregano. Stir and lower heat. Let simmer for about 15 minutes.

While sauce simmers, place chicken thighs in a dry frying pan over medium high heat, skin side down. When skin is crispy flip thighs, turn down heat to medium and cover.

While chicken cooks, finish the sauce. Add cream cheese to the sauce and stir occasionally until cheese is melted and sauce is smooth (except for vegetable chunks, of course). Sprinkle one to two teaspoons hot sauce and stir. Taste to confirm there is a tang in the sauce, but not necessarily a strong spiciness. If not enough tang, then add more hot sauce. Simmer for about 15 more minutes.

When chicken is cooked through and juices run clear, remove from heat and let rest. Remove chicken from pan and place on serving dish. Pour sauce over chicken and serve immediately, or serve on individual plates with sauce drizzled over chicken.

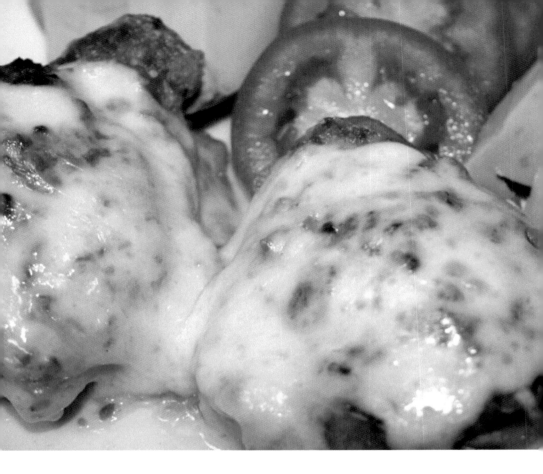

3–4 pound package skinless chicken thighs, or breasts cut
   in strips
1 teaspoon chili powder
1 teaspoon ground cumin
1 teaspoon salt
½ teaspoon ground black pepper
2 cups salsa verde with tomatillo sauce (see Sauce
   section for recipe)
2 cups mozzarella cheese

Chicken Tomatillo

Salsa verde is one of my favorites. Combine it with our staple protein of chicken thighs and it makes for a quick main dish that works for dinner and leftovers. Especially if you use my salsa verde recipe!

Prep Time: 10 minutes

Cook Time: 1 hour (plus 10 minutes cooling)

Servings: 8

In a small bowl combine chili powder, cumin, salt and pepper.
Get your hands dirty and cover chicken with spice mixture, then place in a 9"x13" glass baking dish.
Pour tomatillo sauce over chicken, then top with cheese.
Bake uncovered for 45 minutes to 1 hour, until chicken is cooked through and juices run clear. Let sit for about ten minutes before serving.

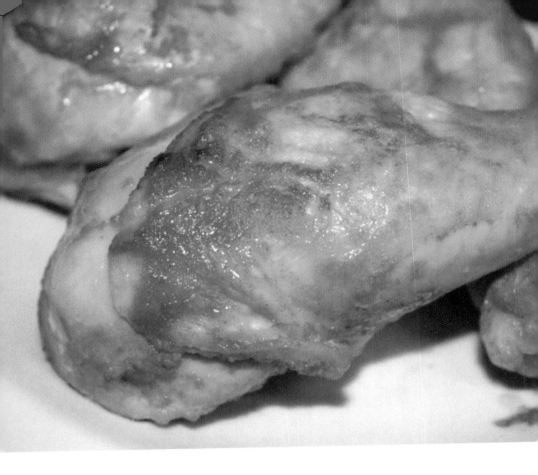

10 chicken legs, skin on
½ cup yellow mustard
¼ cup lemon juice
1 tablespoon Worcestershire sauce
2 teaspoons garlic powder
1 teaspoon onion powder
½ teaspoon turmeric
1 teaspoon salt
Salt and pepper to taste

Lemon Mustard Chicken

I have found mustard to be a great thickener for sauces when flour or cream just don't fit the bill. That is, if you like mustard, which I do. The flavor of these legs reminds me of roasted chicken I had many years ago, which was coated with what I decided was a mustard sauce in a little place I used to frequent in Denver. As often happens, I don't remember the name of the place or the dish, but I remember the flavor.

Prep Time: 15 minutes

Cook Time: 1 hour

Servings: 10

Preheat oven to 375 degrees.
Lightly season the chicken with salt and pepper.
In a 9"x13" baking dish, place seasoned chicken.
In a medium bowl, whisk together mustard, lemon juice, Worcestershire sauce, garlic, onion, turmeric, and salt.
Drizzle sauce over chicken, making sure the tops of all the chicken legs are covered.
Bake for 45 minutes to one hour, until juices run clear.

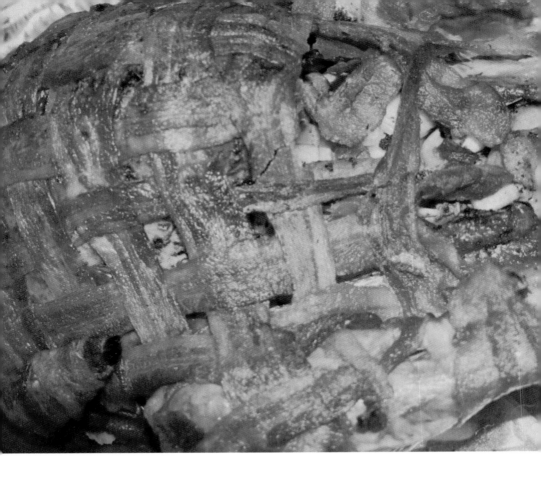

One 15-pound turkey
1 cup fresh parsley leaves
½ cup fresh tarragon leaves
½ cup fresh sage leaves
¼ cup rosemary leaves
10 cloves garlic, peeled and crushed
½ cups olive oil
4 cups chopped vegetable mixture, including carrots, celery,
  onion and garlic
3 pounds bacon, sliced into thin strips

Bacon-Wrapped Turkey

It was fun to do the bacon wrapping and watch the bacon get dark and crispy. Instead of having the typical crispy turkey skin to eat, we had a blanket of bacon. The skin kind of melted into the meat, and became part of the bacon. I am not sure how it happened, but the results were very satisfying.

The bird was stuffed with carrots, celery, onion, garlic and the herb combination that turned out wonderfully doing it's job to infuse the turkey meat.

Prep Time: 1 hour 40 minutes (includes bacon crosshatch and 1 hour chilling)

Cook Time: 4 hours

Servings: 12

Wash the turkey inside and out and pat dry. Place in refrigerator for at least an hour uncovered to chill.

Preheat the oven to 500 degrees.

Mix together the herbs, minced garlic, and olive oil to make a paste. Rub the paste in the cavity and underneath the skin of the breasts of the turkey, carefully so you do not tear the skin.

Fill the cavity with the vegetable mixture, and place in a roasting pan. Add 1 - 2 cups of water in the roasting pan, so there is about ¼ inch of water, then roast the turkey in the oven for 30 minutes.

While the turkey roasts prepare the cross hatch of bacon. Take two pieces of wax or parchment paper, about two feet long each. Create the cross hatch by alternating bacon pieces into two separate one foot by one foot sections, weaving the bacon like a basket.

After the turkey finishes the first half hour of cooking, remove the turkey and pan from the oven and reduce the oven temperature tho 350 degrees. Move the turkey to a surface where juices can drain and be retained, like a carving board or another roasting pan. Drain any additional liquid out of the roasting pan to be used for the final cooking cycle.

Into the final roasting pan, flip one of the cross hatch sections and flatten it out. Place the turkey on top, then flip the second cross hatch on top of the turkey. It is now time to wrap the turkey in bacon.

Between the wings and legs connect the cross hatch edges from the top and bottom as much as reasonably possible. Wrap the remaining exposed skin on the wings and legs with bacon strips, in addition to the top and bottom cross hatch sections. Make sure to cover all the meat and skin. Add a few more pieces on the top and bottom of the cross hatch pattern, if needed, to cover all surfaces of the turkey.

Insert a meat thermometer in the thickest part of one turkey breast. Put the turkey back in the oven and continue to cook for about 20 minutes per pound (about three hours total for 15 pounds, which includes the high temperature period) until an internal thermometer temperature reaches 160 degrees.

Remove turkey from the oven and let rest for about twenty minutes in the roasting pan. To serve, remove the contents of the cavity and place the turkey on a serving or cutting platter. Depending on how you want to present the turkey, the bacon can be removed and chopped up, served as a topping for turkey portions. It can also be carved along with the turkey, as the top portion will be crispy and crumble onto random slices.

Our family tends to serve the turkey carved, so there is a bowl of dark meat pieces on the bone (legs, thighs, wings) and a platter of the carved white meat breast. Removing and chopping the bacon as a condiment works well with this approach. It is also dramatic to carve the turkey at the table with the bacon left on, which means there will be crumbles distributed. Regardless of the serving approach the meat should be moist and tender, ready to be enjoyed!

BEEF

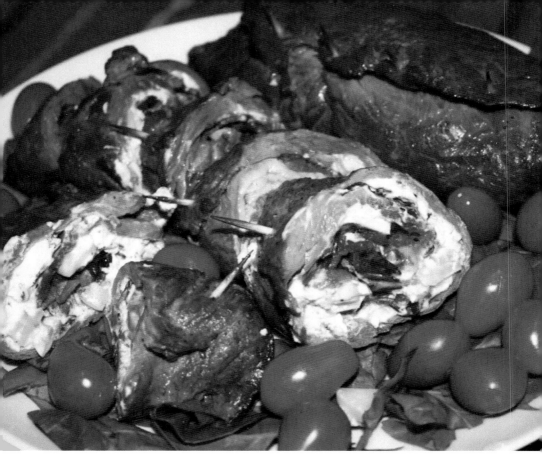

2 pieces flank steak (1½ - 2 pounds total)
8 ounces bacon
½ cup red onion, finely chopped
4 garlic cloves, sliced
4 - 5 ounces goat cheese
1 tablespoon fresh oregano leaves, coarsely chopped
8 ounces fresh baby spinach leaves
8 - 12 wooden toothpicks

Stuffed Flank Steak

Flank steak, also known as skirt steak, used to be cheap. It was a slightly tougher piece of meat that could be marinated and grilled or broiled, cut up and served south Texas style as fajitas. It still can, but the cheapness is gone. I don't know what happened. Maybe, like chicken wings, it got popular and so the price hiked. Did price hike because of demand, or the mere fact the price was higher, so demand increased? The point here is I have turned the once cheap fajita meat into a fancy looking main dish that went POW!

Of course, anything with goat cheese tickles my fancy, but the cheese combined with the steak resulted in a tangy, juicy roll. I made a couple and ended up freezing one, and I discovered it froze well, too! Double POW! You can still make old, reliable fajitas with flank steak, but if you want to get a little fancier, you definitely can!

Prep Time: 25 minutes

Cook Time: 30 minutes

Servings: 4

Preheat oven to 400 degrees.

Slice bacon into ¼ inch long strips.

In a medium skillet over medium heat, cook bacon until it begins to release fat. Add onion and garlic and continuing to cook until garlic slices begin to brown. Transfer bacon, onion, and garlic to paper towel to soak up extra grease.

Lightly salt and pepper the steak. Place steak between two layers of cling wrap. With a tenderizing mallet or side of a regular hammer, flatten steak until about ¼ inch thick. Remove the top layer of wrap.

Spread the goat cheese on the steak, leaving about ½ inch border around the edges. Make a layer of spinach leaves on top of the cheese. Sprinkle the bacon, garlic, and oregano on top of the spinach. Add another layer of spinach. Sprinkle spinach with a little more salt.

To roll the steak, begin by lifting the long side of the steak, pull the steak off the wrap and begin curling it over the spinach. Continue rolling it, squeezing slightly to keep the roll an even size along the length. When completely rolled, place the seam facing up. Impale the roll every inch along the seam with toothpicks. If it is thin on the ends, fold it over and use a toothpick to seal it so the filling doesn't spill out. Place the roll seam side up in a shallow foil wrapped baking dish or baking sheet.

Bake for 20 minutes. Turn oven temperature down to 350 degrees and cook for 10–30 minutes longer, depending on thickness of steak and desired doneness. The first cooking time should seal the meat. The second cooking time will determine the final doneness, between medium rare and well done.

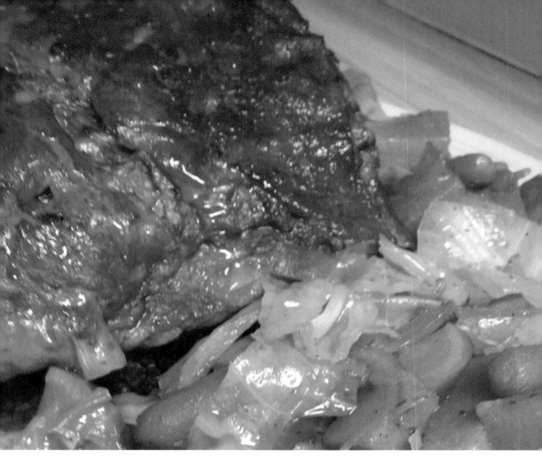

5 pound beef rump roast
3 medium turnips
1 large yellow onion
3 large carrots*
1 cup dry red wine
2 cups beef or vegetable broth
½ cabbage head, roughly chopped
Salt and pepper to taste

*Exclude to reduce carbs/sugars

Beef Roast In Wine

This may make some shudder. I had a craving for beef bourguignon. Knowing I did not have all the ingredients, or time to prep before leaving it to cook accurately to the version by the great Julia Child, I decided to wing it, find a balance, and risk possible imperfection.

So dinner was good, but not traditional. Even if it is not a traditional version, this recipe came out great, allowing for more family time in the evening, and resulting in a mouthwatering dinner.

Prep Time: 20 minutes

Cook Time: 5 hours

Servings: 10

Preheat oven to 300 degrees.

Chop turnips, onion and carrots into bite-sized pieces.

Heat medium oven-proof stock pot or dutch oven to medium high. Season roast generously with salt and pepper. Sear meat on all sides until browned.

Add vegetables and stir, slightly coating them with the browning bits.

Arrange meat so fat side is facing up. Pour wine and broth over meat and vegetables. Cover pot and place in oven. Cook for four hours, leaving it covered the whole time.

Remove pot from oven and uncover. Add cabbage, stir vegetables, trying not to disturb crusty fat layer on top of the meat, and replace cover. Return to oven and cook for one more hour.

Remove from oven, arrange meat and vegetables on serving tray and serve immediately.

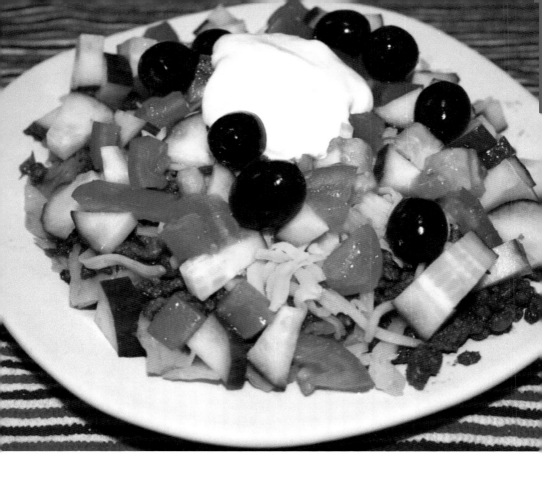

3 - 4 tablespoons bacon grease or other high heat fat
3 tablespoons cumin seeds (optional)
4 garlic cloves, crushed
1 tablespoon red pepper flakes
1 tablespoon Chili powder
1 teaspoon red cayenne powder
1 tablespoon cumin powder
2 chipotle peppers with 1 tablespoon adobo sauce
   (optional)
1 medium onion, chopped
1½ - 2 pounds ground beef
6 - 8 ounces amber or dark beer or beef broth
1 teaspoon salt

Taco Meat

We like it really spicy around here, and often achieve an acceptable level of spice with the wonderfully fresh jalapenos or the smoky version of chipotle peppers in adobo sauce. They are optional, of course, but add a level of flavor we have not found elsewhere, including attempts cumin seeds and various beers. Exclude the stronger flavors in the optional ingredients below if you prefer; otherwise, put it all in and go!

Prep Time: 10 minutes

Cook Time: 40 minutes

Servings: 8

In a large skillet over high heat, add grease. When it is hot, add the cumin seeds, red pepper flakes and optional chipotle peppers. Stir frequently until they begin to darken.

After a few minutes, add the garlic, chili powder, cayenne pepper, cumin powder, and optional adobo sauce. Stir for about a minute until it too darkens. Add the onion and cook until the onions begin to sweat and brown.

Add the ground beef, breaking it up into small pieces while also combining it with the onion and spice mixture. Add ½ teaspoon salt and continue stirring.

When about half the liquid has reduced, about five to eight minutes, add the beer.

Sip on the rest of the beer in the bottle.

Continue cooking over high heat until the liquid reduces again. When most of the liquid is cooked off, turn down to medium heat and continue cooking until most of the liquid is gone. The meat should begin searing.

Drink some more beer.

After searing the meat for about a minute, turn down the heat to low and simmer. Taste, and add more salt to preferred flavor. Let sit with the heat off for about ten minutes before serving.

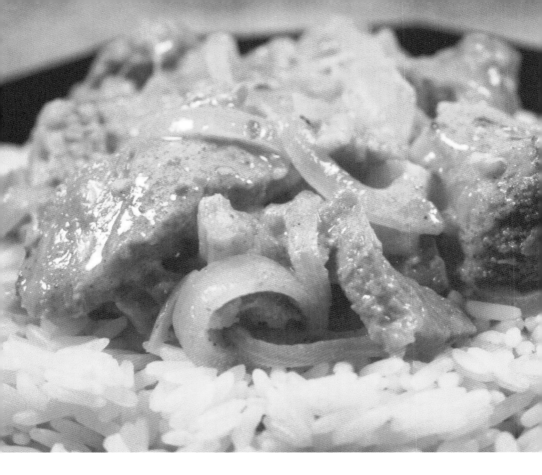

10 - 12 ounces tender cut beef steak, sliced into bite-size strips
3 tablespoons extra virgin olive oil
½ yellow onion, cut julienne
1 pound broccoli, chopped
2 cloves garlic, crushed
1 tablespoon dried chili flakes
2 tablespoons curry powder
1 teaspoon ground ginger
1 cup whole milk (or coconut milk for dairy free)
2 tablespoons lemon juice
½ teaspoons salt

Beef Curry

When my husband took his first bite of this dish I was sitting across the table from him—he smiled and his eyes got big as he quickly reached for his beer. I think I got it spicy enough! I had promised him a spicy dish reminiscent of a favorite he discovered in Anchorage, Alaska, with yellow curry and spinach. It had chicken, but he is more of a beef person, so I changed the focus. The heat can be adjusted by limiting the chili flakes.

Prep Time: 10 minutes

Cook Time: 25 minutes

Servings: 4

Add oil to electric or stovetop wok on medium high heat. When oil is hot, add chili flakes and garlic. As garlic begins to brown, add onions and sauté until they are transparent.

Add lemon juice, curry, ginger, and ½ teaspoon salt. The spices will soak up all the oil and juice pretty quickly. Cook until the color of the mixture changes to a dark brown.

Move onions to the outer edges of the wok. Add beef into the well and toss just until it begins to brown. Toss onion mixture with meat. Lower heat, add milk, and stir until combined.

Add broccoli and cover, lower the heat, and let mixture simmer for about 5 minutes. It is ready when the sauce is hot and the broccoli just tender but still bright green. Serve immediately.

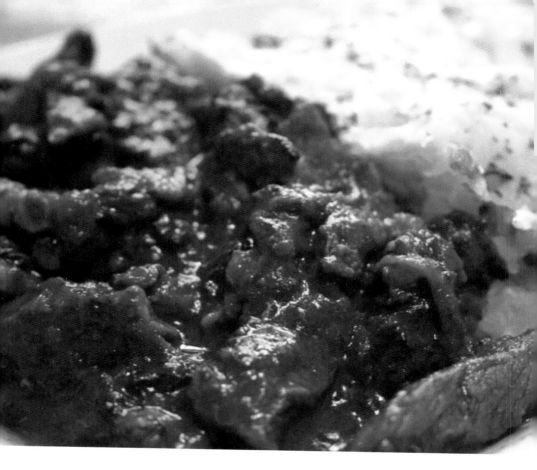

1 tablespoon extra virgin olive oil
½ medium yellow onion, roughly chopped
3 cloves garlic, roughly chopped
2 cups fresh spinach
2 cups tomato puree
½ cup dry red wine
2 teaspoons dried oregano
2 teaspoons dried parsley
1 teaspoon ground thyme
1 dash pure stevia powder (equivalent to 1 teaspoon
  pure cane sugar)
1½ tablespoons butter
1 pound thinly sliced steak
Salt and pepper to taste

Steak In Tomato Spinach Sauce

I prefer rare steak straight off the grill, but if that's not possible, I don't mind baking, or broiling, or smothering it in sauce. I like how the tomato and spinach made the sauce nice and rich. Serve it next to, or on top of, some baked spaghetti squash or zucchini.

Prep Time: 10 minutes

Cook Time: 40 minutes

Servings: 4

Slice steak against the grain into bite-sized pieces, then season generously with salt and pepper. Set aside.

Roughly chop spinach into 1-inch pieces.

In medium pot over medium-high heat, add olive oil. When oil is hot, add onion and garlic. Cook until onion and garlic begin to brown, about two minutes. Add spinach and toss with onion and garlic until most of it wilts, about three minutes. Add tomato puree, oregano, parsley, thyme, tomato, stevia and wine, then stir. Lower heat to simmer, and cook uncovered for about ten minutes until it begins to thicken. Cover sauce and cook for 20–30 more minutes. Set aside.

Five minutes before the simmer time is over heat a shallow sauté pan over high heat. Add the butter. Just before it begins to brown add the meat and toss until coated with butter. Continue tossing until steak is cooked to desired doneness (for me about 3 minutes for medium rare). Remove from heat.

Add the meat to the sauce, stir, and continue simmering for about five minute. Salt to taste.

Serve immediately over spaghetti squash or a side of steamed vegetables.

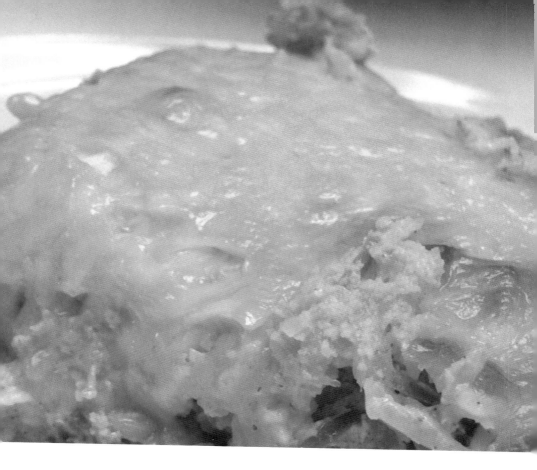

1 large spaghetti squash (or 2½ cups prepared)
1 pound chopped meat (leftover brisket, chicken, pork, etc.)
2 teaspoons garlic powder
1 teaspoon salt
1 cup heavy whipping cream
3 eggs
2 cups Colby jack cheese, shredded

Meaty Squash Bake

I don't know of many meat leftovers that can't be combined and topped with cheese, do you? The nice thing about this recipe is you can cook up some some ground beef for it if you don't have leftovers to manipulate. It freezes well too!

Prep Time: 25 minutes

Cook Time: 50 minutes

Servings: 4

Cut squash in half lengthwise. Remove seeds and strings. In a microwave safe dish place squash halves face down with ½ cup of water. Cover with cling wrap or sealable silicon cover. Microwave for 10 minutes. Let sit in microwave for ten minutes to continue cooking and cool.

Remove squash from microwave and scrape out squash into large bowl.

Preheat oven to 350 degrees.

In a large bowl, stir together squash, garlic powder and salt. Add meat and stir again.

In a small bowl, whisk together eggs and cream. Add cream mixture to squash and meat. Fold until everything is coated with cream mixture.

Pour mixture into 9"×12" baking dish. Sprinkle top with cheese.

Bake for 35 - 45 minutes, until outer edge of cheese begins to brown. Remove from oven and let sit for about ten minutes before serving.

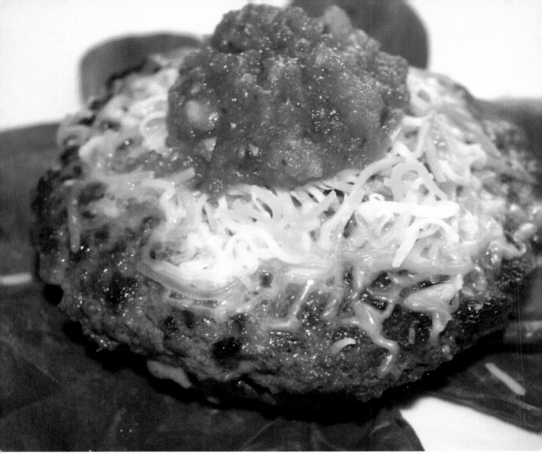

2 pounds ground beef
2 eggs
½ teaspoon salt
¼ teaspoon ground black pepper
1 teaspoon cumin
Dash dried red pepper flakes
1 large avocado
2½ cups shredded co-jack cheese
Salsa for serving (look in the Sauce section of this book for
    recipes)
Fresh spinach or greens and/or buns for serving

Stuffed Burgers

If it can all go on top, why can't some go in the middle, too? In the world of hamburgers, there are a limitless number of topping combinations, and I have tried a lot of them. My go-to combinations are usually the traditional bacon and cheddar, or bleu cheese with mushrooms. I am not a fan of Hawaiian themed burgers—it is my opinion that pineapple is for dessert, not for pizza or burgers. The more exotic burgers with truffles and seafood are okay, but such toppings seem to pair better in a pasta or soup. Although messy, we can cover my burger anytime with spicy queso dip and/or guacamole. Use a bun or not. Either way, a good burger is a messy burger!

Prep Time: 20 minutes

Cook Time: 20 minutes

Servings: 4

Remove avocado meat from skin and roughly chop into small pieces. Set aside.

In a medium bowl, combine together beef, egg, salt, pepper, cumin and pepper flakes.

Divide beef into eight portions, then form portions into thin, equal sized patties. On four of the patties add ¼ cup of the cheese, avocado, and then ¼ cup more of the cheese, leaving about ½ inch of meat around the edges.

Place the other four patties over the loaded ones, then press/form together the edges so there is no seam.

In a frying pan over medium heat, add the olive oil. When oil is hot, add the burgers. Cook for 5–7 minutes on each side, until cooked to desired doneness. The burgers will not take as long as regular burgers to cook because the cheese and avocado will heat up quickly in the middle.

At the last minute, sprinkle the final ½ cup of cheese among the tops of the burgers and cover until melted. Place each burger on an individual serving plate over a bed of greens, and serve immediately.

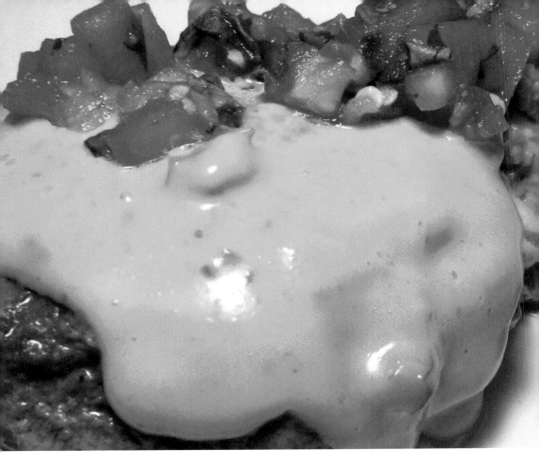

2 pounds ground beef
1 pound chorizo sausage
2 eggs
½ cup fresh cilantro, chopped
3 garlic cloves, crushed
1 teaspoon ancho chile powder
½ teaspoon salt
1 teaspoon ground cumin

Condiments:

1 batch chile con queso (melt horrible chemically
   processed cheese block with a can of tomatoes and
   chiles, some chopped fresh tomatoes and jalapenos)
1 batch salsa (see Sauce section for recipes)
1 batch guacamole (see Appetizer for recipe)

Chorizo Burgers

Since we avoid traditional buns, and I rarely make low carb buns, the variety in our burger-ness relies on combining meats and toppings. Here are some with a spicy flair. Between the pepper and the ancho chile, the burgers definitely left a slow burn in my mouth, and on my lips. They were delicious!

Prep Time: 20 minutes

Cook Time: 15 minutes

Servings: 8

Ensure the queso, salsa, and guacamole are prepared in advance.

For the burgers, combine the eggs, cilantro, garlic, chile powder, salt, and cumin. Whisk together until eggs are combined.

In a large bowl, smush together beef and sausage until they are fully incorporated together.

Add egg mixture and smush some more until eggs, herbs, and spices are well combined.

Form meat mixture into eight large patties.

In a large frying pan over medium high heat, sear one side of the burgers, about five minutes. Flip burgers and sear other side. Reduce heat by half, cover burgers and cook until done, about eight minutes.

When done cooking, immediately place burgers on individual serving plates and top with queso and guacamole. Sprinkle with salsa and serve.

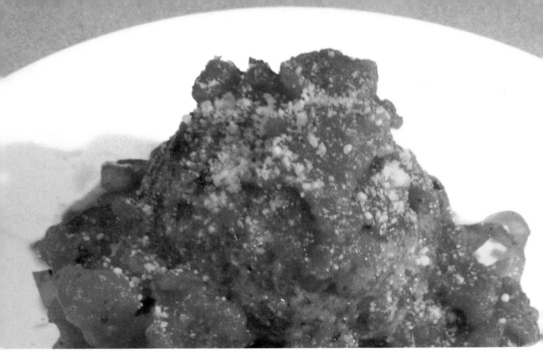

Balls

1 pound ground beef
¾ pound ground hot Italian sausage
2 eggs, lightly whisked
1 tablespoon dried oregano leaves
2 teaspoons dried basil leaves
1 teaspoon dried parsley leaves
2 teaspoons garlic powder
1 teaspoon salt
¾ cup Parmesan cheese, finely grated, plus more for serving
1 tablespoon olive oil

Onions

1 large sweet onion, sliced into thin rings
1 cup water

Sauce

1½ cups diced tomatoes
1 teaspoon dried oregano leaves
1 teaspoon dried basil leaves
½ teaspoon garlic powder

Ultimate Meatballs

These meatballs are massive and arrogant and a little scary. I maxed out my hands trying to form them into balls, but it worked! Making them on the stovetop worked pretty well, allowing for browning on all sides. The stove was busy though, with making the sauce and onions and meatballs! The sweet of the sautéed onions balanced out the bite of the meatballs and tartness of the tomatoes.

Prep Time: 40 minutes (includes chilling, onions and sauce simultaneously)

Cook Time: 30 minutes

Servings: 8

MEATBALLS: In a small bowl, combine the spices—oregano, basil, parsley, garlic, salt, and cheese. Set aside. In a large bowl, squish together the ground beef and sausage until mixed up well. Add the eggs and spice mix, making sure all the meat is coated and spices distributed. Refrigerate at least 30 minutes, or until sauce and onions are ready.

ONIONS: To prepare the onions, heat a deep pan over medium high heat until hot. It should be dry. Add the onion rings and let sit for a minute without stirring until they begin to brown and sweat. Stir them every minute or two, allowing the onions to brown more. When onions are about half browned, add ½ cup water and scrape the bottom of the pan. Stir and continue cooking until the liquid cooks away. Add another ½ cup of water, scrape the bottom of the pan, stir, and continue cooking until the liquid again cooks away. Sprinkle with salt to taste. Turn off the heat, and cover until time to serve.

SAUCE: While onions cook, prepare sauce. In a small sauce pan over medium heat combine tomatoes, oregano, basil, garlic, salt and pepper. Stir. When bubbly, turn temperature down to low and simmer, covered, for at least 30 minutes. Salt to taste

When it's time to cook the meatballs, remove meat mixture from refrigerator (can be prepared the day before). Heat large frying pan to medium high heat and add oil. Form meat into eight huge meatballs, placing them immediately into the hot pan. When forming the balls, make sure to press the meat together firmly and roll it around in your hands to make them as round as possible. As one side of each meatball browns, gently turn them to another side. Repeat this a few times so three or four sides are a bit brown.

Lower heat, cover, and cook until meatballs are cooked through, about 20 minutes. Depending on your stove, you may need to move them around during the cooking time to prevent the outsides from overcooking.

To serve, arrange a layer of onion on the plate, add a meatball or two, and top with the tomato sauce and Parmesan cheese. Serve immediately.

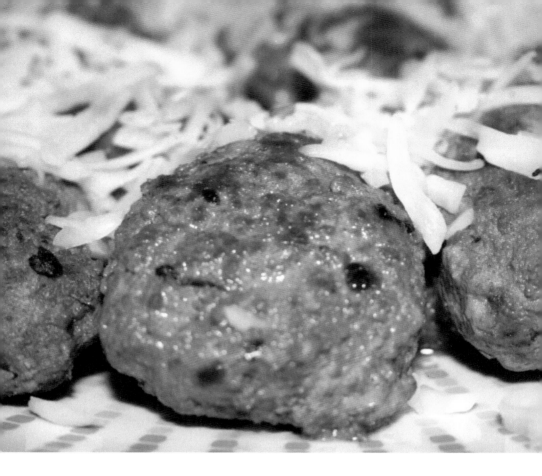

2 pounds ground beef
½ small onion, diced
4 garlic cloves, diced
1 egg
2 tablespoons butter
2 teaspoons dried red chile flakes
1 teaspoon ground paprika
2 teaspoons dried basil
1 teaspoon salt
1 cup pepper jack cheese

Smoky Meat Pucks

These pucks are a result of compromise—some people wanted meatballs and others wanted burgers. My attempt to comply with all the requests resulted in small burgers. I loved the smoky flavor coming from the chile flakes and paprika.

Prep Time: 20 minutes

Cook Time: 10 minutes

Servings: 10

In a medium frying pan, melt 1 tablespoon of butter over medium high heat. Add onion and garlic. Cook until it is all a dark, caramelized color. Set aside.

In a bowl, place the ground beef, egg and spices. Add the onions and garlic. Use your hands to blend together all the ingredients. Form meat into about 10 thick, small 2" patties.

Melt the remaining butter in a frying pan over medium high heat. Cook the patties to desired doneness—about five minutes, including flipping, for medium. Plate and sprinkle with cheese before serving, either with a side of vegetables or slider-type burger buns.

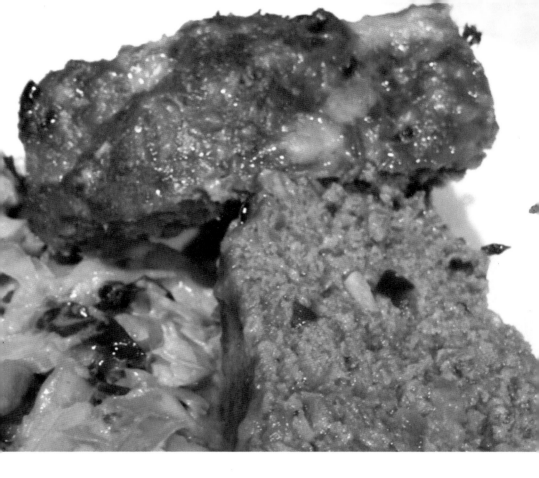

1½ pounds ground beef

2 tablespoons avocado oil

1 poblano pepper, chopped, seeds removed

½ medium onion, finely chopped

3 stalks celery, finely chopped

4 cloves garlic, finely chopped

1 tablespoon chili powder (adjust amount to preferred spiciness)

2 teaspoons ground cumin

2 teaspoons cumin seeds

½ cup fresh cilantro, roughly chopped

¼ cup fresh parsley, roughly chopped

2 cups grated cheese (suggest cheddar or colby/Monterey Jack mixture)

Salt to taste

Spicy Poblano Meatloaf

I remember when I was a kid I would make fun of the meatloaf my mom made. Not because it did not taste good; it was awesome. It was just a thing. I was not alone in this form of entertainment–my dad and brother joined in too. They liked the loaf just like me and always had seconds.

I am still not sure why we decided to make fun of it, but one day mom had a little too much of the kidding and declared she would not make meatloaf again. She was serious. I don't remember ever having her meatloaf again after that night. Regardless of the edge over which we pushed mom, I still consider meatloaf a childhood comfort food.

An important thing about meatloaf is not to forget the smushing of ingredients with hands. There is no way to properly combine ingredients without using hands. Don't even consider excluding this step. Don't.

Prep Time: 30 minutes

Cook time: 1 hour (plus 10 minutes cooling)

Servings: 6

Preheat oven to 375 degrees.

Add avocado oil to medium frying pan over medium high heat. When oil is hot, add pepper, onion, celery, cumin seeds, and garlic. Sprinkle generously with salt. Stir and cook until soft and browning begins.

Add the chili powder, cumin, cilantro, and parsley and stir. Continue cooking until liquid is reduced and some browning begins. Set aside mixture and let cool slightly.

In a large bowl, add ground beef, eggs, and cheese. With your hands, mix together the three ingredients until well combined. Add cooked mixture and combine well. Load the meat into a 9"x9" square baking dish and press down firmly.

Place in oven and bake for one hour, until the loaf separates from edges of pan and the cheese bubbles up and begins to brown. Remove pan from oven and let cool for about ten minutes, letting the bubbling liquid settle. Serve with a vegetable side.

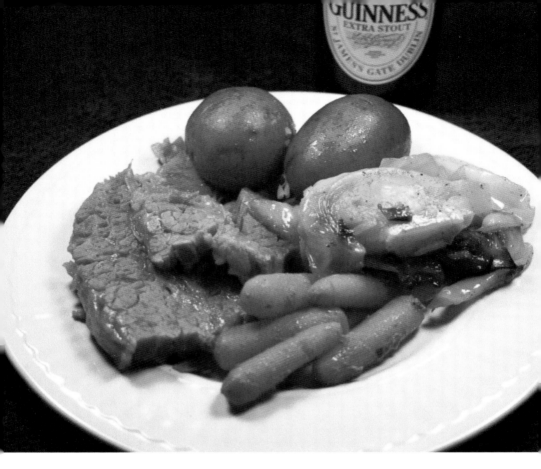

4 pounds corned beef
2 large carrots, cut into 2-inch sticks
5 - 7 small potatoes or turnips, halved
   (optional)
4 cups water
1 tablespoon pickling spices
1 small head cabbage
Salt and pepper to taste

Corned Beef And Cabbage

"May the road rise to meet you and the wind be always at your back. May the sun shine warm upon your face and the rain fall softly on your fields. And until we meet again may God hold you in the palm of his hand."
-Unknown

I included directions for cooking the cabbage separately (boiling or sautéing), because it does not always fit with the meat and veggies in the crock pot. You might think a six-quart crock pot would be big enough, but not for us! We like our cabbage in bulk!

Prep Time: 10 minutes

Cook Time: 8 hours

Servings: 8

Pour water and pickling spices into 5-6 quart crock pot. Add beef and cook on high for two hours, then turn to low. Add carrots and potatoes, and cook for 4 to 6 more hours until vegetables are soft.

Cut cabbage in half and remove core. Slice halves lengthwise into wedges–enough to fit in one layer in a large pan with cover.

To boil cabbage: about 45 minutes before meat is done, pour enough water in the pan until it is about ½ inch deep, including one to two cups of juice from the crock pot. Add some salt and bring to a boil. Place cabbage wedges in the water, lower heat to simmer, and cover. Cook for about 25 minutes until tender. Gently remove from pan with a long spatula, trying to keep the wedges intact. Salt and pepper to taste.

To sauté cabbage: about 30 minutes before meat is done, heat large pan to medium high and add about 3 tablespoons butter. When melted, spread it around the pan. Place wedges in pan and cook until browning begins. Flip wedges gently and let brown again. Cover pan and lower heat until cabbage is soft. Gently remove from pan to a serving dish, trying to keep the wedges intact.

Serve the corned beef and vegetables with spicy brown mustard and creamy horseradish.

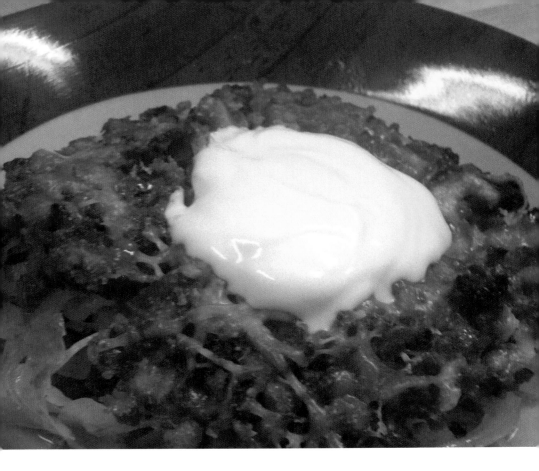

1 small head cabbage, finely shredded
1 medium carrot
1 small yellow onion
5 cloves garlic
3 tablespoons extra virgin olive oil
20 fresh basil leaves
⅓ cup fresh oregano leaves
½ cup fresh thyme leaves
1 cup fresh parsley sprigs
2 pounds ground beef
2 cups diced tomatoes
1 cup tomato sauce
Salt and ground black pepper to taste
1 teaspoon ground nutmeg
1 cup grated Parmesan/asiago/romano cheese
Sour cream (optional for serving)

Deconstructed Cabbage Rolls

Although the ingredients are not seasonally limited, I always consider cabbage rolls to be an autumn dish. They are a baked, one dish meal that freezes and reheats well.

I think the key to this dish is the well shredded cabbage. It cooked faster than larger pieces or fully rolled cabbage rolls. Also, the small cabbage pieces helped soak up all the wonderful flavor of the fresh garden herbs I used, as well as the joyful combination of beef and tomatoes in the alternating layers.

Prep Time: 45 minutes (includes sauté)

Cook Time: 1 hour (plus 10 minutes cooling)

Servings: 8

Chop onion, carrot, and garlic into small pieces.

Roll the basil, oregano, thyme, and parsley leaves into a small roll. With a sharp knife, slice the herb roll. Cross-chop the herbs again, until the oils are released.

In a large iron skillet over medium high heat, add the olive oil. When the oil is hot, add the carrot, onion, and garlic. Cook for about two minutes, until the onions begin to turn transparent and brown. Add the chopped herbs and stir, cooking for another two to three minutes.

Clear the vegetable mixture from the center of the skillet. Add the ground beef and break it up, folding in the vegetables as the beef pieces get smaller. When the meat is broken up into small pieces and beginning to brown, add the diced tomatoes and tomato sauce. Let bubble and cook, stirring every few minutes, until the liquid reduces by half, about five to eight minutes. Turn heat down to medium and simmer for another five minutes. Salt and pepper generously to taste.

Preheat oven to 350 degrees.

In a 9"x13" baking dish, place half of the shredded cabbage into an even layer. Sprinkle with salt, pepper, and ½ teaspoon of ground nutmeg. Add a layer of the meat mixture, making sure half of it is left for another layer. Add a second and final layer of cabbage, again sprinkling with salt, pepper and the rest of the nutmeg. Add the second and final layer of meat, covering all the cabbage.

Sprinkle the cheese mixture on top of the meat layer.

Place in preheated oven on the top shelf. Bake for 30 minutes. Check the top of the casserole, making sure it is not browning too quickly—if it is, place it on the middle or lower shelf. If is is barely brown or not at all, leave it on the top shelf.

Bake for 30 more minutes. Remove from oven and let sit for 10 minutes before serving with sour cream or creme fraiche.

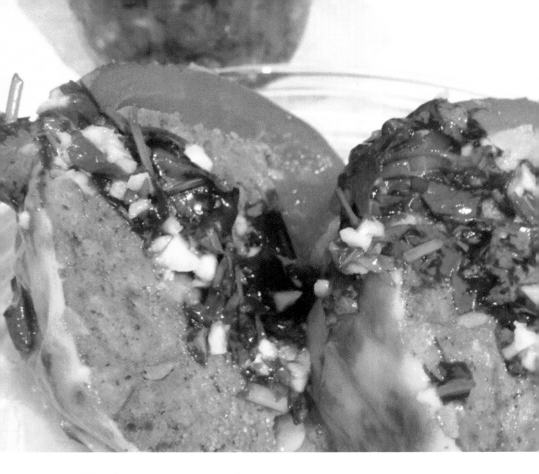

6 bell peppers, any color
½ large onion, finely chopped
½ pound ground beef
½ pound ground sausage
1 egg
1 cup Colby/Monterey Jack cheese, grated
1 teaspoon ground cumin
5 garlic cloves, chopped
½ teaspoon salt
½ teaspoon ground black pepper
½ teaspoon red chile flakes
1 cup beer or beef broth
5 - 6 slices Monterey Jack cheese
Salt to taste
1 batch chimichurri or guacamole (see Sauces sections for
   recipes)

Stuffed Bell Peppers

I used to never like stuffed peppers. They were often overcooked, filled with flavorless rice, and they often left me hungry. When I first made stuffed peppers for myself, I decided to eliminate the unsavory elements. These peppers offer you a lively, substantial, satisfying meal.

Prep Time: 20 minutes

Cook Time: 1 hour 15 minutes

Servings: 6

Remove top of each pepper and remove pulp and seeds from inside. Rinse, shake out excess water and place in 8 x 11 inch baking dish.

Divide onions equally among the peppers by dropping them into the bottom of each. Sprinkle onions with salt.

In a large bowl combine beef, sausage, egg, grated cheese, cumin, garlic, salt, black pepper and chile flakes. Using your hands is the best method.

Firmly press the meat mixture into each pepper until it is level with the top. Arrange the peppers evenly spaced in the baking dish. Carefully pour the beer or broth in the bottom of the dish. Bake for 45 minutes.

Place a slice of cheese on top of each pepper. Return to oven and bake for an additional 20 minutes, until peppers are soft and cheese begins to brown. Remove from oven and let cool for about ten minutes.

I suggest serving drizzled with chimichurri or guacamole.

PORK AND SEAFOOD

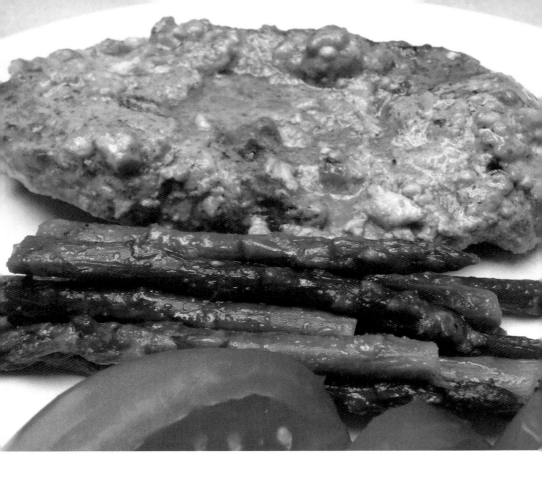

2 tablespoons extra virgin olive oil
6 thin cut pork chops (with or without bone)
1 lemon, juiced with meat retained
1 lime, juiced with meat retained
1 clove garlic, minced
Salt and pepper to taste
1 cup crumbled feta cheese
½ cup heavy whipping cream

Tangy Feta Pork Chops

Just like chicken, pork is quick and easy to make, so the challenge is adding variety to the flavors surrounding it. A lot of my chicken and pork recipes are interchangeable, like this one, because both proteins represent mild flavored bases. Another easy way for me to make pork chops is to sear, make sauce, pour it on chops and bake for a bit. I call it SSPB–Sear Sauce Pour Bake.

The prep is quick, and if forces beyond my control delay dinner, then letting them sit in a turned off oven after they are done cooking does no damage. I know such things NEVER happen to anybody else, but if it ever may happen to me, this is the type of dish I'll make.

Prep Time: 10 minutes

Cook Time: 45 minutes

Servings: 6

Preheat oven to 350 degrees.

With kitchen scissors or a knife, make a ½ inch slit in the curved fat edge of each pork chop, towards the center. This step will help prevent the chops from curling up on the edges while they cook. Generously season pork chops with salt and pepper.

Place three chops in a large frying pan over high heat, cooking until downward facing side is seared, about two minutes. Flip chops and repeat searing. Remove chops to 9"×13" baking dish. Repeat searing with remaining three chops.

Turn heat to medium low. Add lemon and lime juice to pork drippings in the pan, scraping brown bits from bottom. Add feta and cream. Stir until sauce is bubbly, about 3-4 minutes. Pour sauce over pork chops.

Cover baking dish with foil and bake for 20 minutes, until pork is cooked through (internal temperature should be at least 145 degrees) and juices run clear. Chops can be served immediately, or left in oven with heat turned off to keep warm until served.

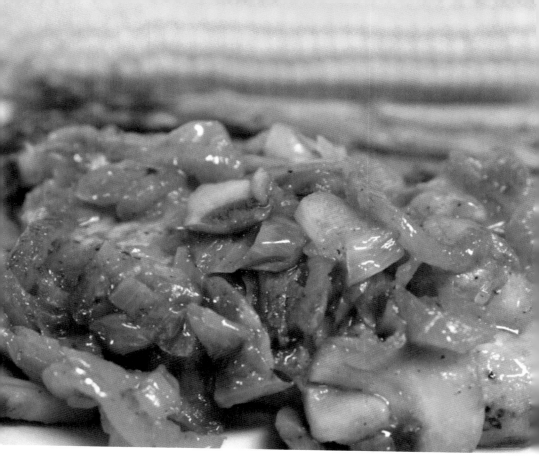

8 boneless pork chops, ½-inch thick
3 cloves garlic, crushed
1 tablespoon dried thyme leaves
2 teaspoons onion powder
½ teaspoon chili powder
1 teaspoon salt
½ teaspoon ground black pepper
¼ cup lime juice
2 tablespoons extra virgin olive oil
1 medium yellow onion, sliced into thin rings
8 ounces white button mushrooms, sliced thin
½ cup water
Salt and Pepper to taste
1 tablespoon butter

Smothered Pork Chops

Pork chops are my friend and foe. It is so easy to overcook them, yet undercooking is just plain unappealing. The perfect balance is having the pink just recently disappearing and the chops beginning to firm up.

My solution in most cases is to smother them. It often does not matter what is used to smother, but just to have something to go with the juicy chops. Sometimes I use some homemade applesauce (try it, I promise you will like applesauce and pork), other times it may be a smoky, spicy chipotle sauce. This recipe uses onions and mushrooms, with a hint of lime.

Prep Time: 35 minutes (includes marinating time)

Cook Time: 45 minutes

Servings: 8

In a resealable bag combine garlic, thyme, onion powder, chili powder, salt, black pepper, lime juice, and olive oil. Shake the bag until the marinade ingredients are mixed up. Add the pork chops. Seal the bag, letting out as much air as possible. Spread out the chops in the bag until they are all one layer and thoroughly coated by the marinade. Let sit for at least 30 minutes, turning over at least once.

While the chops marinate, make the smother. In a dry medium sauté pan over medium high heat, add the onions and sprinkle with salt. Toss sparingly until they begin to sweat and begin to brown, about five minutes. When there is some caramelizing on the bottom of the pan, add ¼ cup of water. Scrape the bottom of the pan and stir until the caramelizing dilutes in the water and begins to make a sauce. It will all turn a golden brown. Continue cooking over medium high heat until the liquid mostly evaporates, probably another five minutes or so.

When most of the liquid has evaporated and there is more caramelizing on the bottom of the pan, add the remaining ¼ cup of water, scrape the bottom of the pan, and continue cooking until the liquid begins to evaporate again.

Add the mushrooms and a little salt and pepper. When the mushrooms begin to sweat and soften, turn the heat down and let simmer until the sauce is reduced by half. Add the butter and stir until it is completely melted. Set aside and keep warm for serving.

Remove pork chops from the marinade and gently pat dry to remove some of the marinade liquid. In a large dry frying pan over high heat, add the chops and cook on each side for about a minute to sear. If there is extra liquid it may take a few minutes longer. When both sides are browned, cover the pan and reduce heat. The pork chops will release more liquid and keep them moist while the pork cooks completely. When the pork is well done (at least 145 degrees), turn off heat and keep warm until time to serve.

To serve, place a pork chop on the plate, drizzle a little juice from the bottom of the pan over the chop, then top with the onion and mushroom mixture. Serve immediately.

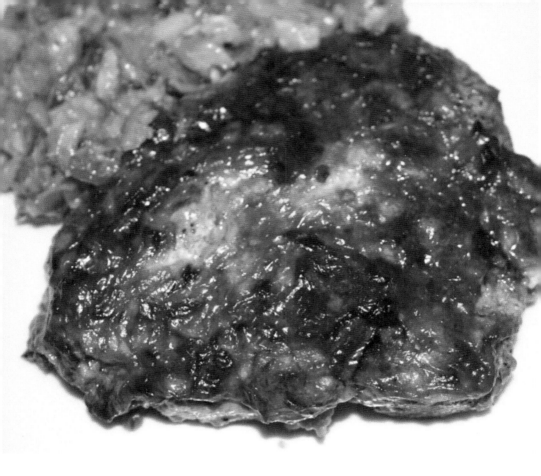

1 tablespoon olive oil
4 bone-in, 1-inch thick pork chops
1 small can chipotle peppers in adobo sauce*
½ cup mayonnaise (in Sauces)
1 teaspoon lime juice
Salt and Pepper to taste

*This recipe also works with a small can of green chiles, which will not look as dramatic but will be less spicy. Also, make sure wheat is not included in the list of ingredients for chipotle in adobo, if you are sensitive, for some brands include wheat.

Chipotle Pork Chops

These pork chops are not only pretty, but they pack quite a flavor punch! We often use chipotle peppers in adobo for barbecue sauce or with red meat, but not so much with pork. It was a nice change to feature the peppers with the milder pork.

Prep Time: 10 minutes

Cook Time: 45 minutes

Servings: 4

Season pork chops with salt and pepper.

Place oil in pan on stovetop over medium high heat. Add pork chops and sear on both sides. They will not be cooked through. Remove from heat.

Preheat oven to 375 degrees.

In a small bowl, place about three peppers and half the adobo sauce from the can. With a fork and sharp knife cut peppers into small pieces (you can also put peppers and sauce in a food processor to chop). Add mayonnaise and lime juice. Stir until well blended.

Place pork chops in a baking dish. Spread sauce over chops. Place in oven, uncovered, and bake until meat is cooked through to at least 145 degrees, about 30 minutes. Serve with something soothing, like a salad or guacamole, to help soften the spiciness.

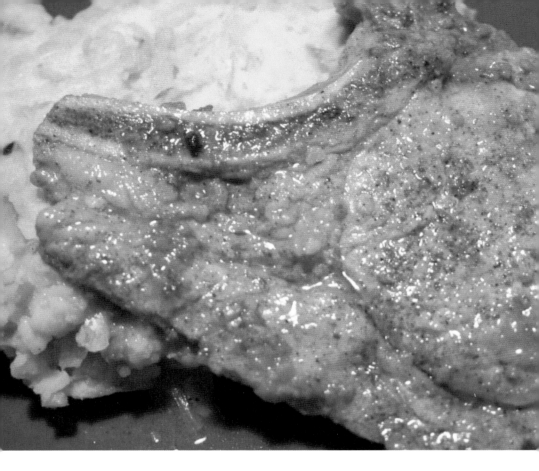

4 thin cut bone-in pork chops
3 tablespoons olive oil
1 tablespoon stone ground mustard
2 tablespoons lime juice
2 tablespoons apple cider vinegar
2 cloves garlic, chopped
Salt and Pepper to taste

Mustard Cider Pork Chops

I enjoy making simply prepared dishes just as much as complicated ones. Many more modern Irish dishes combine sweet and savory to complement meats, which is what I did here. These chops go great with cabbage or mashed cauliflower.

Prep Time: 5 minutes

Cook Time: 25 minutes

Servings: 4

Make two slits in the meat of each pork chop, 2 - 3 inches apart along the fat strip, cutting towards the bone. This step will help prevent the chops from curling up on the edges while they cook. Season chops with salt and pepper.

Heat a large skillet over medium-high heat. Add oil. When hot, add garlic and cook until it begins to brown. Add mustard, honey, and lime juice. Stir until combined and hot.

Place pork chops in the pan, press down a bit, then flip, allowing both sides of the chops to be covered with sauce. Cook on each side for about 3 minutes until seared. Decrease heat to medium-low and cover pan, cooking until pork is cooked through (at least 145 degrees), about ten minutes.

Serve immediately.

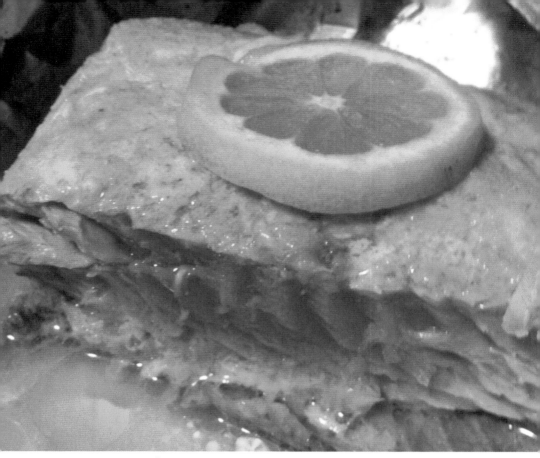

Poached Salmon

Depending on my salmon craving, I vary the preparation–do I want tart, or sweet and spicy, or maybe traditional dill with citrus? I should have called this recipe 'variations on a salmon' because each time I make it the ingredients vary. I am going to discipline myself for the time being and make sure you have a good base recipe, then list some variations that give the salmon subtly different flavors.

Even if you can't find the freshest or never frozen salmon, this recipe still works on any piece, as long as it is completely thawed.

Prep Time: 20 minutes

Cook Time: 25 minutes

Servings: 6

Basic Poached Salmon

1 - 2 pound fresh salmon fillet
1 lemon
4 tablespoons vinegar (apple cider, red wine or white wine)
2 tablespoons butter or extra virgin olive oil
Salt to taste
Additional ingredients from the variations below

Preheat oven to 350 degrees.

On a shallow baking sheet, place a piece of aluminum foil. The foil should be twice the length of the pan plus about four inches– with the center of the foil in the center of the pan. The salmon will be completely enclosed in the foil, like a steam pocket.

Salt the skin side of the fillet. Place the salmon fillet skin side down in the middle of the foil and bend up the foil edges, so the liquid does not leak out. Drizzle juice from half the lemon over the fish, followed by drizzling vinegar. Sprinkle salt over fillet lightly.

Add any additional ingredients from the variations below. For variations with liquid ingredients, I recommend mixing them all together before adding to the fish.

When all ingredients have been added to the salmon, fold over the edges of the foil and seal into a pouch so no fish is exposed. Bake for 20 - 25 minutes until desired doneness. It is better to undercook than overcook, so check the middle of the thickest part of the fillet. Cook for a few minutes longer if needed. Remember, if left outside the oven covered up, the salmon will continue to cook in the steaming pocket.

Variations:

1 tablespoon fresh dill
1 clove garlic, finely minced
½ lemon thinly sliced into discs to arrange on top of salmon

Or

2 teaspoons ginger, freshly grated
2 tablespoons gluten free soy sauce or coconut aminos

Or

3 tablespoons fresh cilantro leaves
½ teaspoon chili powder
1 teaspoon ground cumin
½ lemon thinly sliced into discs to arrange on top of salmon

Or

1 tablespoon honey
1 teaspoon ground cinnamon
2 teaspoons ginger, freshly grated
½ lemon thinly sliced into discs to arrange on top of salmon

Or

½ cup mayonnaise (in Sauces)
1 teaspoon garlic powder
1 teaspoon onion powder

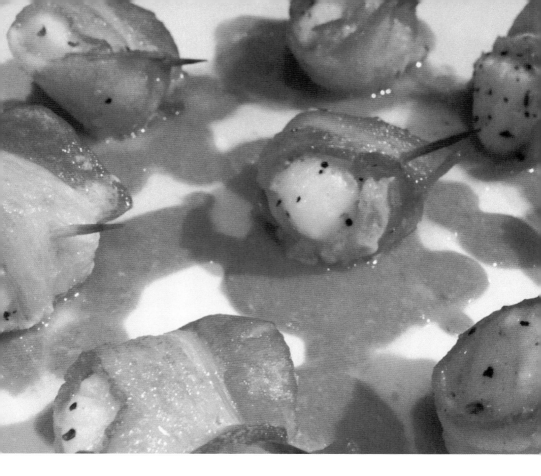

8 large scallops (at least 1" diameter raw)
4 slices bacon, cut in half*
8 round toothpicks
Salt and pepper to taste

Spicy Cocktail Sauce

1 tablespoon tomato paste
1½ tablespoon raw horseradish, grated
¼ cup lemon juice

Bacon-Wrapped Scallops

I broiled these scallops since the little guys are easy to overcook and quick cooking works well with the broiler. I was tempted to do more seasoning, but decided to keep it simple. I was not disappointed. These were so easy to make at home and delicious!

Prep Time: 10 minutes

Cook Time: 10 minutes

Servings: 4

Preheat oven on low broil.

Lightly sprinkle scallops with salt and pepper. Wrap a piece of bacon around a scallop, overlapping the edges. Secure the bacon with a toothpick, pushing it through both sides of the scallop. Repeat with all scallops.

Place scallops in a shallow baking pan. Position oven rack in the middle of the oven, at least 8 inches below the broiler. Place scallops in oven. Broil for about ten minutes, making sure not to overcook the scallops.

If you only have one broiler setting, assume it is high and reduce cooking time to 5-7 minutes, watching carefully–a few more minutes may be needed, depending on broiler heat. The bacon may smoke a bit.

While the scallops cook, make the spicy cocktail sauce: whisk together the paste, horseradish and juice until well blended. Sprinkle sauce on serving dish.

Place scallops on the serving plate with cocktail sauce immediately after removing from the oven.

*This recipe will result in cooked bacon, but not fully crispy all around. If you prefer crispier bacon you can partially cook the slices in advance, before wrapping the scallops.

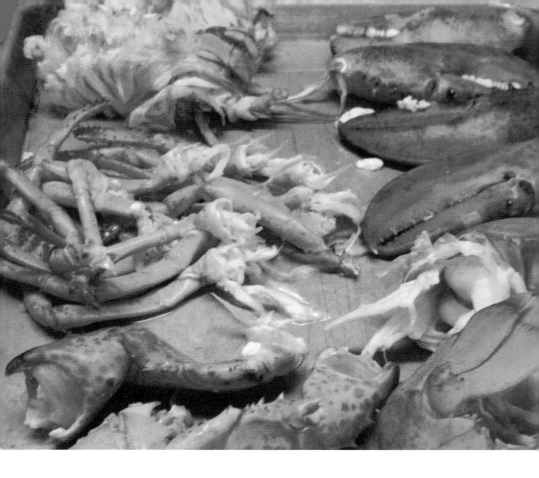

1 pound unsalted butter
2 lemons
2 lobsters, 1½-2 pounds each
2 - 3 gallons water
2 bay leaves
Salt to taste

Boiled Lobster
with Clarified Butter

A most despidsed dish to me is overcooked, dried out lobster. It is sad that such a delicious creature gets so abused for our sake. Not the eating of lobster; I am fine with doing that, but the overcooking of it. For that reason I do not often order it in restaurants. Maybe it is unfair to assume they will screw it up, but it is what I do. My parents were the same way. They would not eat them in restaurants, but buy them alive the afternoon they planned on cooking, and leave the suckers in the sink to wait. When I was young and short, I would peek over the edge of the counter and see them moving around, with their claws bound in rubber bands. According to my mom, one of those claws once came towards me and I freaked out. Apparently it was hilarious. I am not sure if I thought so at the time.

If you have never prepared fresh, live lobster, from crawling to consuming, you are missing out. The meat cannot be compared to previously frozen tails or the disguising of it in a lobster roll or dip. It is pure, sweet, meaty heaven. The reason for keeping them alive until right before cooking is to preserve them as long as possible. Like all shellfish, they begin to break down (organs and all) immediately upon death, so delaying death as long as possible is the healthiest, safest way to prepare them.

If you have never used clarified butter, you may wonder why is it important to use it, instead of just melting butter right out of the fridge. It is my opinion, and that of many others, that if the butter is not clarified, with a hint of lemon, the butter will take over the flavor of the lobster instead of enhancing it, and leave a greasy film in the mouth. Leftover clarified butter is a great fat for cooking other things, so none of it will go to waste. It is the foundation of butter without the milk solids and water, so it has a high smoking point for cooking other foods and contributes a wonderful butteriness to whatever you cook.

Prep Time: 35 minutes (4 hours in advance) plus 20 minutes

Cook Time: 15 minutes

Servings: 2-4

About four hours before cooking the lobster, the butter needs to be prepared. In a medium sauté pan over medium low heat, add butter and zest from one lemon. Heat until butter is melted and steaming. Remove from heat and pour butter through a sieve to remove zest. Let butter sit for 20-30 minutes. Skim off fat layer that forms on top. Pour the remaining butter into a measuring cup or clear glass bowl. Place in refrigerator and let chill for at least four hours.

In a large stock pot, add enough water to cover both lobsters, and squeeze in lemon juice from one lemon. Drop in lemon rinds and bay leaves. Bring water to a rolling boil. Remove rubber bands from lobster claws. Drop lobsters into the boiling water, head and claws first. Cover and boil for 15 minutes, until shells are red.

While the lobsters cook, you should complete the clarified butter. Remove butter from refrigerator and scoop out the yellow, clarified portion from the top, leaving separate the white, watery portion (water and milk solids). Heat clarified butter over medium heat until melted and steamy.

Remove lobsters from water and set on a tray to cool. Serve whole or remove edible meat from shells and serve on a platter. If you need more information about extracting meat from a lobster, I suggest you search online. There are plenty of step by step instructions and videos that are very helpful.

Serve with the clarified butter, and eat by dipping each bite into the butter, or drizzling plain lemon juice over the bites.

BEVERAGES

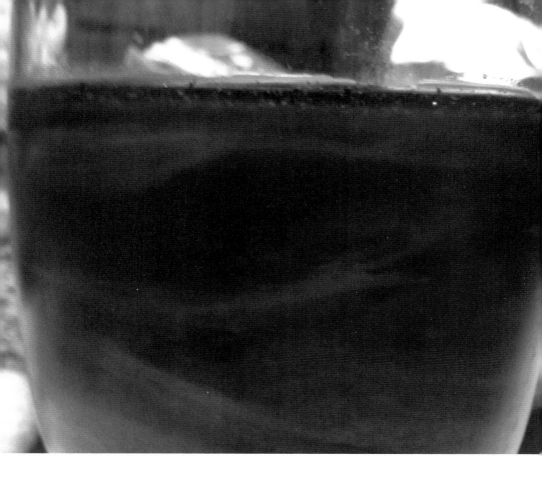

½ cup dark roasted coffee, coarsely ground
4 cups cold water

Optional flavors for serving:

Heavy cream
Half and half
Cinnamon
Nutmeg
Sweetener

Cold Brew Coffee

My favorite caffeine boost in the summer is cold brewed coffee. It is easy and delicious and does not require a coffee maker. I like mine with a little cinnamon and cream. I use dark roasted coffee and there is no bitterness. Just deep, toasty flavors that only weaken slightly as the ice melts. Of course, there are endless possibilities when it comes to doctoring up the final product with spices and creams and sweeteners. Deep in the summer I lean towards just a splash of cream, then as fall nears I go heavier on the cinnamon and nutmeg, before I finally turn to hot coffee as the summer wind is replaced with cool autumn breezes.

Prep Time: 5 minutes

Cook time: 24 hours chilling

Serving: 4

In a quart sized jar* with screw lid add water and coffee. Screw lid on tightly and shake. Place in refrigerator for 24 hours. Leaving it for more than a day will not hurt it. Strain liquid into another jar or bowl, through a sieve with coffee filter lining it. Rinse jar and return coffee to it. Store in refrigerator. To serve, fill your serving cup about ½ way with coffee and add ice until glass is filled. If the coffee is too strong for your taste, add a bit of water.

If you like, stir into the coffee about 1 - 2 tablespoons of heavy cream, a dash of cinnamon, and any sweetener or other spices–the way I like it–or have it straight, which is delicious, too!

*Cold brewing can also be done in a french press. It may be a smaller volume, but makes the filtering process easier. Just keep the 8:1 water to coffee ratio, and it works out the same as using a jar. When you use a french press, you need only to put it in the fridge with the plunger up, or leave the plunger out and cover the top of the press. Before serving, gently press down the plunger to filter the coffee.

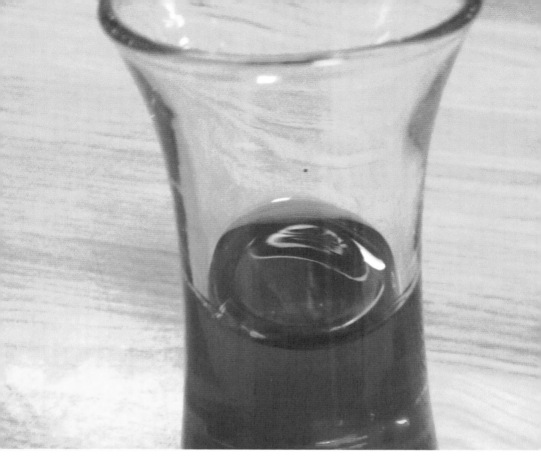

Approach One:

1.75 liter bottle whiskey
5 cinnamon sticks
1 teaspoon cayenne pepper powder
½ teaspoon pure stevia powder

Approach Two:

1.75 liter bottle whiskey
2 cinnamon sticks
¼ teaspoon cayenne pepper powder
12 - 15 sugar free cinnamon candies, broken up
   small enough to be dropped into the bottle

Cinnamon Whiskey

The problem with flavored liquors is the mystery surrounding the content of the added flavoring. Do they have fillers? Exactly how much sugar do they use? What other chemicals are in that bottle of goodness? Such beverages do not have ingredient lists on the bottles or the websites of companies, so a lot of digging goes into actually figuring out what is in them.

One of my favorite flavored liquors is cinnamon whiskey. I can tell from just one sip that, among other things, sugar is definitely added. My attempts at creating my own cinnamon whiskey, so I knew what was in it, resulted in two versions. They both have sweeteners, because, honestly, some sweet is why I like it.

The first approach is ideal because it is sweetened with stevia and satisfies my cinnamon hankering. The second approach, using sugar free candies with the sweetener of your choice (or sugary candy if you like) makes the end result very closely match the candy sweetness inherent in commercial cinnamon whiskeys.

Regardless of the approach you use, the end result is a pretty, festive red whiskey with a lovely, spicy bite to it!

Prep Time: 5 minutes

Cook Time: 2 days mulling with shaking 2-3 times daily

Servings: 55

Remove ¼ cup whiskey from the bottle. Add cinnamon, pepper, and candies/stevia to bottle. Replace top on bottle. Let whiskey sit for at least two days, shaking it two to three times a day. Shake before each use. Serve neat, on the rocks, or with mixers as usual.

The last cup of the whiskey in the bottle will have more sediment and be slightly bitter, so I recommend using it for mixed drinks instead of neat or on the rocks.

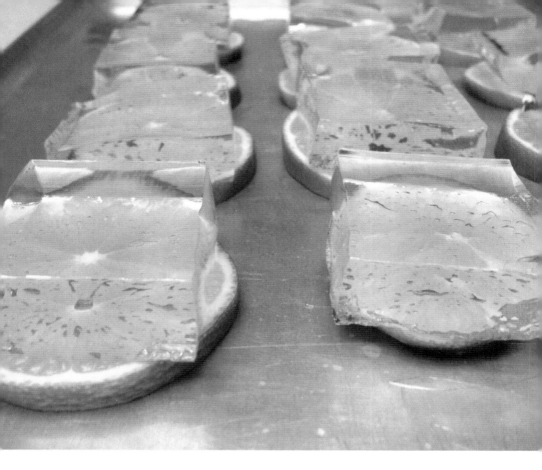

3 cups tonic water

½ teaspoon pure stevia powder (equivalent to ⅓ cup
   pure cane sugar)

6 teaspoons unflavored gelatin (Knox brand usually has
   2 teaspoons per envelope)

1 cup gin

6 - 8 limes, sliced into 6 rounds each

Gin And Tonic Shots

I wanted to have fun with gelatin. I remember summer gelatin fun as a kid–mixing it with whipped cream, making jiggly things that can be picked up, bowls of shiny, wiggly stuff that fell off a spoon. If you look at the flavored gelatin packages in the store, you will find either sugar or aspartame in them. Really? Aspartame in a product you are expected to mix with boiling liquid? Have they read any of the information about the stuff and the dangers of heating it?? I will get off the podium/verge of preaching and move on…

My favorite cocktail of all time is a gin and tonic. It took a couple of tries to get the liquor/non-liquor liquid ratio right, but I figured it out. I do agree that they are not a substitute for slowly sipping a tall gin and tonic on the rocks during a hot summer evening, but they were a fun variation to liven up a dinner party.

I remember first seeing the lime presentation in a magazine a billion years ago (well, maybe ten); unfortunately I do not remember where, so crediting it must remain a mystery. Happy summer to you!

Prep Time: 30 minutes

Cook Time: Chill overnight

Servings: 36-50

Heat 2 cups of tonic water and stevia until boiling. While liquid boils, add final cup of tonic water into a medium bowl. Sprinkle the gelatin over it, letting it sit for one minute. Add hot liquid to bowl and stir until gelatin is completely dissolved. Add gin and stir. Pour mixture into a 9"×9" baking dish, or pour into approximately 50 mini paper cups/mini cupcake papers, or split between both methods. If using mini cupcake papers, I suggest arranging them in mini cupcake pans, for the liquid will seep through. Refrigerate at least overnight.

To serve from the dish, cut shots into 1 to 1½ inch cubes with a sharp knife, removing from the dish with a thin, flexible spatula. Place squares on lime rounds to serve. If using paper or cupcake cups, gently peel away paper and invert them on lime rounds. To eat, tip shot into mouth, then with your teeth fold the lime round in half and bite down, releasing juices to mix with the shot.

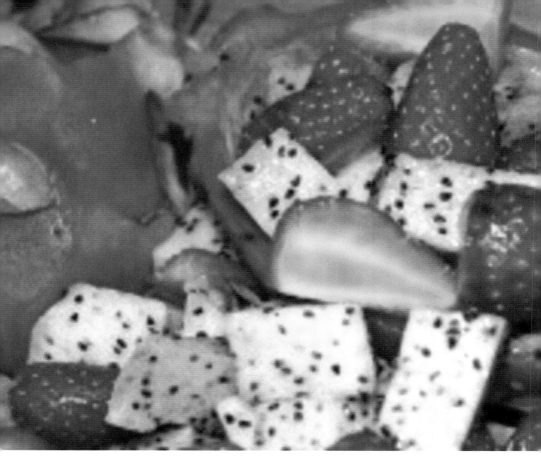

Prep Time: 10 minutes

Cook Time: 0

Servings: 2 each salad and cocktail

Dragon Fruit Frenzy

Dragon Fruit is the funkiest fruit I know. It is bright and crazy on the outside and and a neutral black, white and mild on the inside. It kinda tastes like kiwi fruit, but unlike the skin of the kiwi, you should shy away from eating the thick pink skin of the dragon fruit. With a single dragon fruit you can make two simple recipes–a fruit salad and a rather odd looking cocktail. The meat of the dragon fruit can be sliced or cubed and looks really pretty with brightly colored fruit.

For the cocktail I did a margarita-type drink (I know, blasphemy for the margarita purist), and enjoyed sipping it. With my eyes closed, the cocktail was soft and lovely. With my eyes open, it looked like a gray sludge that tasted soft and lovely. I don't know what to do about the color, but it tasted wonderful.

If you are not a fan of grey frozen cocktails, just double the salad recipe and enjoy!

Salad

    ½ dragon fruit, meat cubed
    1 cup strawberries, quartered
    Squeeze of lime
    ½ shell of dragon fruit

Combine dragon fruit and strawberry pieces. Drizzle with lime juice. Present in the shell of the fruit.

Cocktail

    ½ dragon fruit, meat only
    4 - 6 ounces tequila
    ½ lime, juiced
    ¼ teaspoon pure stevia powder
    6 cubes ice

Add stevia and remaining ingredients to blender. Blend on high until ice is broken up. The sweetness of the fruit can vary, so taste the cocktail and add more stevia to preferred sweetness. Serve immediately.

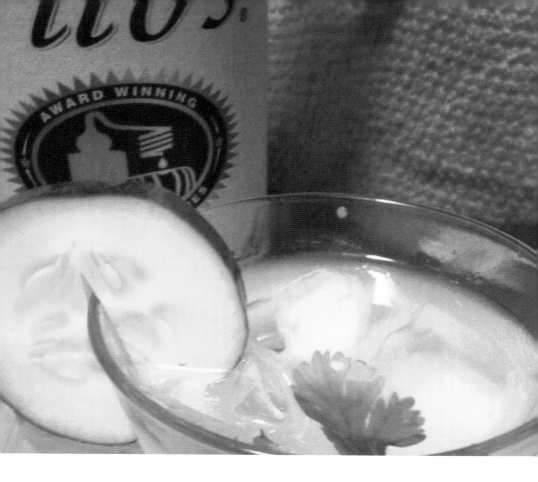

½ cup chopped cucumber, seeds removed
Small handful of fresh cilantro
2 ounces vodka
1 lime (or 2 key limes), juiced
Pinch of pure stevia powder
Ice
¼ to ½ cup Seltzer water or club soda (optional)

Cucumber Cilantro Cooler

Cilantro is best when fresh leaves and stems are used. I like storing it in a jar with water to keep it fresh as long as possible.

This cocktail comes out fresh, tangy and perfect for a hot, humid summer evening. I also made a version with tequila, which is also very enjoyable, so if you are not a vodka drinker, try it with your liquor of choice.

Prep Time: 8 minutes

Cook Time: 0

Servings: 1

Add chopped cucumber to a cocktail shaker, along with a large handful of cilantro leaves. Muddle well, and then add vodka, lime juice, stevia, and ice to almost fill the shaker. Shake well for twenty seconds, then strain into a lowball glass filled with ice.

If you want to make the cocktail a little less powerful, strain it into a taller glass and top with a splash of seltzer and ice, then stir quickly.

Garnish with a wheel of cucumber and a sprig of cilantro. Sip sip sip!

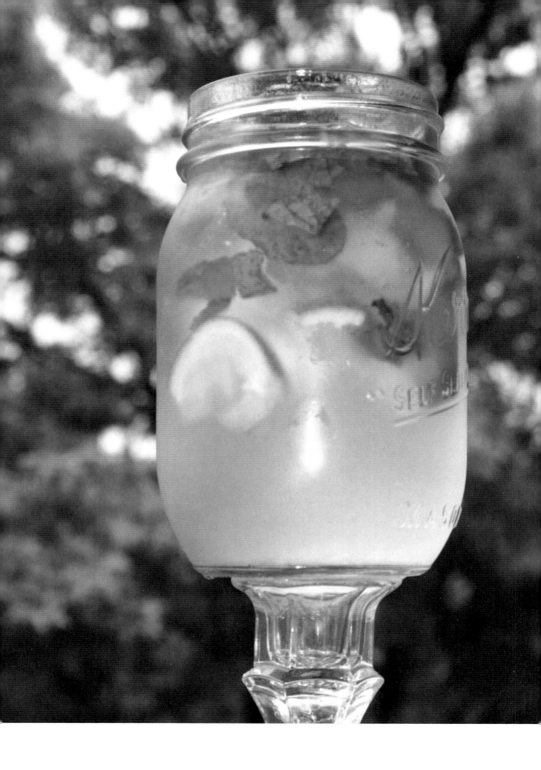

Mojito

The first true mojito I had was made by a neighbor many years ago. She prepared a big pitcher of them as cocktails at the beginning of a dinner party. When poured over ice and muddled mint, it was a welcome refreshment on a warm Virginia evening. Here is a lower carbohydrate version that is still light and refreshing.

Prep Time: 5 minutes

Cook Time: 0

Servings: 1

½ lime, divided into thirds
2 - 3 sprigs fresh mint
¼ teaspoon pure stevia powder
2 ounces rum
8 - 10 ounces club soda
Ice

In a tall glass, add lime pieces, squeezed, and half the mint leaves, gently torn or muddled. Add sweetener and rum. Stir mixture with teaspoon until sweetener is dissolved. Add soda, and then ice, to fill the glass. Imbibe. Relax.

AFTERWORD

AS I MENTIONED in my first cookbook, there might be a second. Here it is! I also mentioned that the second, like the first, would reflect our life. Here it is!

The reality of eating differently from the typical American diet is that you will occasionally, or often, find yourself in a situation where you may or may not find much to eat. You will find people who question why you are not eating (I'm fasting!) or why you don't have a pile of mashed potatoes on your plate (yikes!) or why won't you just dip your veggies in the ranch dip (seed oils!).

On the one hand, you can try to explain it. On the other hand, you can bring a dish to the potluck you can actually eat. If you are hosting a meal, you can make and serve a healthy, delicious meal that everyone can enjoy.

This book is about those gatherings where you want to focus on the family and friends, but can sometimes be derailed by food and nutrition discussions. *Our* family and friends sometimes don't know what to do with us, but one thing they cannot dispute is that the food is good, and they leave full and satisfied, with leftovers.

We continue on our imperfect path of grain and sugar free eating. The little blurbs at the start of the recipes are to try and show that we don't float through life, but move forward in it.

The first cookbook has given me personally a lot of joy, helping me meet many who have bought it, and giving me the opportunity to sign it for them. I am now doubling my joy being at able to offer up this second effort of love, further sharing parts of my life and loves, for they often intertwine.

Again, I hope my efforts will help make your journey easier. My desire is to enhance your food journey, both personally and functionally. It is an old mantra, but you are what you eat! May this book help your contents!